Successful
Losers

I thank my husband for the unconditional love and support he has dedicated to me since the day we met.

To our sons, Gabrieland Teodor, who have given me the best gift of all - the privilege of being their mother.

TABLE OF CONTENTS

Introduction

Why you should read this book before going on any more diets

Have you ever wondered why some people manage to lose weight and keep it off, while others are constantly going on diet after diet with no results? In fact, a stunning four out of five dieters regain their starting weight within two short years [1]. How is it that some people manage to look and feel great while eating all of their favorite foods - or end up with a fantastic body without ever going to the gym? Who are these people? What do they do differently? What are their secrets?

With these questions in mind, I started an obsessive search for Successful Losers – normal people like you and me who have achieved the permanent weight loss we all aspire to – and set out to discover what makes these people remarkable and different from the rest of us. What is it that they do or think that make them succeed in maintaining a healthy body weight where most of us fail?

This book is the result of that search and my own research as a scientist in nutrition – a fascinating journey through the medical literature and hundreds of hours of interviews with real life Successful Losers about the life changing habits that make all the difference. It turns out that there are real secrets for successful weight loss – and that these really work! By learning from and emulating the Successful Losers, you too will find the formula for sustainable weight loss, healthy eating, and the path to your ideal body. When it comes to permanent, healthy weight loss and – more important – weight maintenance, this is the most important book you will ever read. Not only does it contain all that you need to know to become a Successful Loser yourself – it also reveals that the way to a healthy body does not go through dieting, short-term fixes and miracle cures.

Why should you listen to me?

Before becoming a certified dietitian with a Master's degree in nutrition, currently in pursuit of a PhD in clinical nutrition, I was myself an uncontrolled eater in a permanent fight with the scales. Out of simple self-preservation, I have always been fascinated by why we eat what we eat, and how our food affects our lives. Throughout my career, I have worked with obese, anorectic, bulimic and plain fat people – and what they all have in common is their constant struggle to make lasting changes.

As a teenager, I was happily fat until I was about fourteen years old. That is when I bought into the current ideal of a perfect body – and started to aspire to all the promised happiness this new body would bring. I lost 40 pounds by dieting and became a slim young woman. All of a sudden, I was skinny. Boys started noticing me, the new clothes I bought actually fit and food suddenly did not seem to threaten me anymore. Indeed, it seemed like I had it all figured out, and that my new, skinny body really brought happiness and a new sense of control to my life. Encouraged by this, I started to obsessively learn about more and more ways of dieting, eating, and staying fit. Soon, I found myself totally emerged in this new way of living. Everything I ate had to be low in fat, low in calories and sugar-free. Every single calorie had to be counted, recorded and – most importantly – burnt. My exercise routine went from two mandatory hours per week at school to a demanding regimen performed for 3 hours a day, five days a week, and including everything from swimming to lifting weights. All carefully planned out and designed to burn the maximum amount of calories and exercise every muscle in my body!

A normal weekday used to look like this: I woke up at 6:30 am and had a powder protein shake for breakfast (mixed with water instead of milk – a glass of milk was way too caloric). Then I would go to school (often, I missed the school bus on purpose forcing me to walk some 30 minutes to get to school). At lunch time, I would eat my own packed lunch, usually consisting of either a chicken salad or a tuna sandwich (needless to say, no dressing or mayonnaise). After school, I would go for swimming class or running before heading directly home to do my homework. Then it was time for the gym for my sacred daily workout session – but before that I might allow myself an apple or a handful of strawberries. For dinner, I would have another powder protein shake – only this time with milk!

Come the weekend, I suddenly changed into another person. All my discipline broke down, and I would tune out and obsessively indulge in all of the forbidden foods that I did not allow myself during the rest of the week. In fact, I had an out of control eating disorder, stuffing myself to the point that I had to throw up afterwards. So, you might say, how bad is a little binging if you can still look great in a bikini? And how come no one noticed what was going on? Well, to the first question I answer very, very bad and to the second that having an abnormal relationship to food is almost considered the norm amongst young women in our society! On the surface, there seems to be little to worry about. I was a good girl after all, with grades that were above average, never tasting alcohol, smoking or doing drugs. And there is nothing wrong about taking care of one's appearance, right? Even if it means bleeding stomach ulcers, rotting teeth and a total lack of self-esteem?

After countless sessions with a therapist, I realized that I was trying to deny a big and important part of myself. In fear of becoming fat again – and thereby losing the only thing that I thought made me attractive to others – I went to unhealthy extremes. In fact, after studying and researching nutrition, I now realize that I committed the terribly common mistake of embarking on an unsustainable, unrealistic and dangerous lifestyle change that was damaging rather than healthy for my body. In fact, many of the restrictive miracle diets sold to you can lead to eating disorders – and none of them are sustainable over the long term [2, 3]!

After escaping from my personal eating hell, I have now maintained my current weight for over 15 years and through two pregnancies. I have done this by changing unhealthy habits into healthy ones and making sure that I have my facts straight – something I can safely say applies to every Successful Loser! In fact, the more I learnt about the food and our bodies the more I wanted to share that knowledge with others. Helping people to lose weight in a healthy and sustainable way has become a passion, and my life project.

Who is this book for?

Just to be clear, you definitely do not have to have a PhD in nutrition to develop healthy eating habits and manage to lose weight – not even a high school diploma! Sustainable weight loss and healthy living depend on discipline and common sense – and most Successful Losers do not have any special training. What they do have, however, is an overwhelming desire to achieve their goals and thereby enjoy a healthier and more fulfilling life. You can learn from other people's experience – and by emulating their empowering habits you can help yourself to succeed. This book is about learning things that really work from such role models – but more important than the stories that you will read are the attitudes behind the stories. Successful Losers take charge of their own lives, believe in themselves and in their ability to overcome life's challenges – and if they do not possess stamina and determination to start with, they develop it along the way. So join me for an insider's view of these select individuals, whose habits and attitudes will be revealed in this book – along with how you can use them to become a Successful Loser yourself!

This book is aimed at readers who want to improve their health and quality of life through losing weight and staying slim – regardless of your gender, color, physical appearance or education level. I believe that you will find this book useful if you answer yes to any one of the following questions:

- ❖ Do I want to lose weight without dieting?
- ❖ Have I managed to lose weight before, only to gain it all back again soon after?

- ❖ Have I managed to lose weight and now want to learn how to keep the weight off?
- ❖ Do I believe that my weight negatively impacts my life?
- ❖ Do I want to have a body that does more and looks better than the one I currently have?
- ❖ Do I believe in practical solutions to transform my lifestyle into a healthy one, one step at a time – no miracle cures or 15-day diets?
- ❖ Do I want to help a loved one to lose weight – or to maintain an achieved weight loss?

Finally, even if much of the advice given in this book can be applied to the whole family, it is aimed at adult readers. Also, if you suffer from any chronic disease that requires a special diet or frequent medical attention, I advise you to consult with your dietitian or doctor before attempting any changes to your lifestyle.

How to use this book

The book is divided into three parts. In **Part 1 - How to get started**, you will learn about who the Successful Losers are and what they can teach you, the many reasons for why you eat what you eat, and the danger overweight poses to your health. Most importantly, you will discover if you are ready to become a Successful Loser yourself, and, if so, how to set attainable and realistic goals that really work to effect change.

In **Part 2 - Secrets of Successful Losers**, I will reveal the secrets that every Successful Loser knows – secrets that if you adopt them will help you to lose weight and stay slim for life. You will learn what makes Successful Losers so successful, and how to become a Successful Loser yourself! And more, at the end of every chapter, you will find practical tips and exercises that will help you to unlock your own secret formula for attaining your goals.

In **Part 3 - Tricks of the trade – what do expert dietitians know that you don't!** You will learn why calories are talked about so much, how not all calories are created equal, and that food is a drug. Last but not least, you will learn that to err is human – but that to persist in erring is just stupid!

This is a hands-on book. Learning the secrets of Successful Losers is only the first step – putting them into practice is rather more important. That is why Successful Losers is full of practical tips and exercises that teach you how to put your knowledge into action. I strongly believe that if you are really willing to think and act like the Successful Losers in this book, you will become a Successful Loser too!

Part I

How to get started

[1]

Who are the Successful Losers?

Successful Losers are not super-humans blessed with tremendous powers that are only available to them. They are usually not luckier than average, they have not won the genetic lottery or made a deal with the devil. In fact, they are just regular folks like you and me! At this point, you may be thinking: "yeah right, if they were like me they would weigh as much as I do". And you are right! There is one fundamental difference – and it is so important that I have written this book about it. People who successfully lose weight and keep it off for good are better at one thing and one thing only. Read on to find out what that thing is!

Weight loss and, especially, weight maintenance is a very complicated business that depends on changing your lifestyle rather than just changing one single habit. Science shows that Successful Losers usually adopt five or more healthy habits while those who do not lose weight or end up gaining the weight back, usually make far fewer positive changes to their lifestyles [4-6]. If you are in the latter group, don't despair! When you improve one area of your life this positive change usually makes further changes easier as well. For example, as you start eating a healthier diet you are more likely to start exercising, quit smoking and decrease your consumption of alcoholic beverages. Thus, many small changes maintained overtime ultimately lead to a better health and a hotter body. As they say – even a long journey begins with one small step. Contrary to many diet books out there that promise miracle weight loss overnight, I find impossible to claim that any single change leads to immediate weight loss and works better than all others. In fact, the "average" Successful Losers looks very much like this:

They make up their minds to finally lose weight after careful consideration, and then immediately take measurable steps. They also remain committed to losing weight and keep this focus until they reach their desired weight. To get there, they lead an active life with more leisure time spent doing fun outdoor activities (such as, cycling, playing sports or walking) and less time on sedentary activities (like watching TV or surfing the internet). Even after achieving their ideal weight the Successful Loser manages to keep their new healthy habits. They monitor their eating habits, and feel in control over them. Usually their food intake is regular, including breakfast, lunch and dinner, with a few snacks in between. Healthy foods are chosen over unhealthy high-caloric foods. Sometimes, even the most Successful Loser slips up and ends up going back to their old ways – but when this happens they handle their setback in a constructive way without blowing things out of proportion and feeling like a failure. Also, Successful Losers are confident in their ability to achieve their goals – they know that they are in charge of their lives and consequently do not blame other people or circumstances for their disappointments. And more, the life of Successful Losers are usually stable, with less stressful events, and they choose to spend their time with people who also live a healthy lifestyle. Successful Losers know that they are unique – and because of this they tailor realistic lifestyle solutions that fit with the rest of their life [4-6]. Successful Losers report that during their change process, they not only managed to alter their lifestyle, but also – and more importantly they first underwent a change in mind-set that drove them to change their entire unhealthy approach to life.

Typically, these individuals go from seeing weight loss as a cosmetic need that ought to be squeezed in between other pressing commitments, to a deeper and more honest awareness of what their life means to them and why they want to continue to enjoy it for a long time to come. From being mere victims of chance their new attitude told them that they were in control. Consistent in my reports and scientific studies of lasting weight loss is a conscious shift that makes it possible for the individual to be more honest with themselves. So instead of expending time and effort on keeping up appearances or wishing for miracles, most of my interviewees reported realizing that to change their bad habits they actually had to work hard – something that they would do for themselves rather than for their family or friends. Also, most of those interviewed for this book reported realizing halfway or more to their weight-loss goal that losing weight was no longer their main motivation. Instead, successfully changing some aspects of their lives made them conscious of other things that they wanted but had thought impossible to achieve – and made them more ruthless in getting them. Reading this description, I realize that you may be thinking that Successful Losers are actually super-humans (and that their super-power is an out-of-this-world willpower). But one of my main goals with this book is to convince you that this is simply not the case!

Look closer at all of the examples and success stories, and you will realize that Successful Losers do not have exotic and impossible to achieve lifestyle habits to thank for their success. Instead, they are just like you and me but for a realization that they owe it to themselves to live as well and healthily as they can in order to enjoy more of the things they like (yes, even food)!

A good example of a Successful Loser is Mary B., a 41 years old nurse and mother of three. She told me how she managed to lose 53 pounds despite having to work full-time and care for her children. "I never really thought about what I ate until my third pregnancy. I had gained weight during my previous two pregnancies, but never found it very difficult to get back to my pre-pregnancy weight. When I got pregnant for the third time I thought it would be just as easy to lose the extra weight again. Boy, was I wrong! Maybe because I was older this time, I had to work hard to reach my goal – which was to lose the extra 60 pounds I gained during my pregnancy. I started to pay careful attention to what I ate, which I had never done before. Now, I read labels on everything I eat, keep a food diary in order to keep track of my food intake, stop eating my children's leftovers and I also cook more than I did before. On top of all that, I make it a priority to take time out just for myself to exercise (even if it is just 20 minutes most days of the week)".

Successful Losers know that when they reach their coveted weight loss goal, it will not have happened by chance. Nobody loses weight because of luck! Have you ever heard someone say, "Wow, I am so lucky to have lost so much weight" Luck has no place in the journey towards your dream body – and Successful Losers know that. This is evident from a large study [7] by a team of researchers led by Prof. James Hill from the University of Pittsburgh. They asked Successful Losers to rate the difficulty of their successful weight loss. More than half said that their weight loss was either easy or moderately difficult. When asked about the difficulties of weight maintenance, surprisingly 68% reported this also as easy or moderately difficult. These are encouraging finds for those of you who may think that weight loss (and maintenance) is impossible. In fact, when you succeed, I bet that you will answer similarly! As a former fat girl, I must confess that making the change was not easy – but neither was it as difficult as you imagine. It takes motivation, planning, determination, self-confidence, positive thinking, and discipline, just to name a few of the traits needed. Later on this book, you will learn how to acquire and enhance all of these characteristics. The biggest obstacle is to have the guts to pay the price to get the body and the life that you want. Nothing valuable comes easily, but by following the scientifically proven secrets of Successful Losers you will become one!

No one can make you fat but yourself!

Not long ago, the concept of healthy food was virtually unknown. People would eat to survive or, in later times, as a symbol of status – yes, being fat was actually a sign of wealth. After all, not everyone could afford food rich in fat and protein. And with a short lifespan, the negative effects of overweight were hard to notice. Nowadays, for better or worse, things have changed and in most industrialized countries getting enough food is no longer a problem. We have come from striving to get enough food on a daily basis to overeating all too often. We are still obsessed with food, but for all the wrong reasons. So, how did it happen that good food became so trivial in our society that we all eat several times a day without planning or even thinking? How can we not notice that we are consuming more and more? Regardless of hunger or need. Who should we blame for that? In this book we will not focus on who to blame for our generalized overeating as a society, but rather on who is to blame for your overeating – namely you. This book is about what distinguishes the Successful Losers from those of us who spend a lifetime struggling with our weight.

While there are almost infinite reasons why so many people around the world struggle with obesity (we might as well call it the epidemic of modern life!), no one has been able to pin point one specific cause for the obesity epidemic. Yes there are scientific studies that blame our genetic make-up, others that implicate changes in lifestyle, some that point to the widespread availability of junk food, and yet more that find the cause in the sharp decrease in physical activity that comes with office life. And the list goes on and on [8-12]. Personally, I agree that most of these factors, if not all, play a role in our weight and eating choices. But there is one factor that more than any other determines our waistline: our decisions. We are each the result of the hundreds of decisions we make every day. From the time we wake up to the time we go to sleep. We decide if we are going to take a shower or not every morning; the clothes we are going to wear; if we are going to have scrambled eggs in the morning, or milk and cereal, or just skip breakfast all together. We decide if we are going to go to work today, or just hang around the house; we decide if we will go to the gym or go out for dinner instead.

Our decisions shape our lives more than any other factor; they determine who we are – and who we will become. They determine the career we have, the person we have married (or will marry or not marry at all!) and – yes – how healthy and slim our bodies will be. Sure, we can always blame our parents for handing down "bad" genes, or our colleagues at work for bringing all those fatty foods and sharing with us (who can resist FREE and tasty food?), or those evil big food companies that make billions of dollars every year selling us "junk" disguised as food (which we have to buy, right?). Last but definitely not least, let's not forget about our so-called friends – who insist on meeting in our favorite restaurants every time! Life really is not easy for those of us wanting to lose some extra fat around our waists. It even seems like there is a conspiracy to make us embark on a never-ending eating binge. But make no mistake about it, in the end we are all and will always be responsible for the choices we make – and to be healthy and slim is a choice!

"Successful Losers are not born, Successful Losers are made"

Remember, Successful Losers are not born, Successful Losers are made. They certainly are not super-humans living in a separate and perfect world – where there are no temptations, stress, or fast-food restaurants. Like the rest of us they live in a world and a culture filled with all of these things. So, how can they manage to lose weight and stay slim while most of us can only keep dreaming? What triggers our bad food choices? Why do we eat what we eat? Which forces are behind our overeating? In the next chapter, you will learn what really goes on in your body – and mind – when you are about to order a burger with fries.

Chapter 1 in a nutshell

❖ Successful Losers are not different from you or me – they have simply decided to have long and healthy lives.

❖ Healthy weight loss and maintenance is not only possible, but how to achieve these goals is well known to science. And soon you will know too!

❖ Successful Losers go through a stepwise process of change, leading them to adopt a healthy lifestyle. They also develop a changed mind-set that makes their old habits seem alien and going back to them not an option.

❖ Successful Losers are the result of their choices – and so are you. Yes, there are many forces that conspire to make you fat, but in the end you and only you can decide how to live your life.

[2]

Why do you eat what you eat?

You may have heard the saying that you are what you eat (or drink). I think we should instead say that we become what we routinely eat. Not such a big difference you might think. But to me (and millions of overweight people out there) the small words "become" and "routinely" signal a whole lot. What we eat can change from meal to meal, depending on the context. But what we routinely eat is what we eat when we are not thinking – the result of long habit. And our habits now make us routinely eat too poorly and too much – even when we are not hungry! Why is that?

That question is more difficult to answer than you may think! Despite all of the science going on, we still do not have a clear view of the main drivers of food choice. In this chapter, I will discuss some of the most accepted concepts to help you to better understand yourself and your eating behavior. In fact, armed with the knowledge in this book and your own self-awareness, I bet that you will soon be able to tell me why you eat what you eat – and why you keep eating even you are not hungry! Don't get me wrong, I am not advocating another fad diet based on self-denial! Most of us get some amount of pleasure from eating – the more caloric the food, the more pleasure we feel – and this is normal and healthy. This mildly euphoric feeling associated with eating is probably a survival instinct. For most of our existence, we have had to eat whatever food we could find, raise, grow or kill. Food was very precious, while getting enough to eat was the goal of most of what we did. In short, meals were hard to get and boring to chew! Being a picky eater was definitely not an option for our ancestors! Little wonder, then, that we needed the motivation of a small rush to finish our uncooked roots with spoiled raw egg and dirty water! Today, we no longer have this problem. Instead, manufacturing things to eat has moved to factories and producers now spend a lot of time and money on things such as the flavor and texture of our meals, which we often expect to find conveniently packaged at a low cost. Talk about evolution!

Nutrients build and sustain your body

The foods we eat are fundamental sources of energy and nutrients necessary for the functioning of our bodies and for life. Our bodies need energy and nutrients to be able to perform even the most

mundane of tasks, such as breathing, thinking, sitting, and walking. These nutrients are also sources of raw materials used to construct every cell in our body. For the purpose of simplicity, the nutrients in food are divided into 5 groups: carbohydrates, proteins, fats, vitamins and minerals – more on nutrients and nutrition in Chapter 7. Each of these nutrients has a special role in building, repairing and maintaining our bodies and one group cannot be replaced by another. Some key functions also require more than one nutrient, which is why it is important to have a varied diet that includes all nutrient groups. Nowadays, despite an abundance of food never seen before, a healthy diet can still be a challenge – due to lack of time, knowledge or interest.
We eat to live, but many people also live to eat – which is when a lot of the health issues related to overeating start to become big problems. Let's not forget that to most of us, food means so much more than nourishment.

"We eat to live, but many people also live to eat"

Food covers so many aspects of our lives; in most cultures, it is how people socialize, show affection, and deal with their emotions. It is a sign of status and a way to ease loneliness. It allows us to show affection or to punish. With food being such a central and permanent part of our lives, we may as well learn to use it in our favor – to make us happier, stronger and healthier without letting it control us.

Am I hungry or do I just want to eat?

The decision to start or stop eating is a complex process. Hunger is primarily driven by signals originating from the gut and brain. These hunger signals stimulate the seeking out of food and encourage you to eat. Thirty minutes after the start of eating, satiety signals arise from the gut and, in between meals, from the fat tissue and liver. These signals still your hunger by working as tranquilizers on your brain, leading you to stop eating. As you know, pharmacological tranquilizers can be addictive. In the same way, some researchers claim that the "rush" of satiety signals following a need to eat may stimulate some of the same pathways in our brain, can lead to food addiction [13] – more on food addiction in Chapter 8.

With such an intricate system to control eating it is easy to imagine that food was once scarce so that we needed a lot of motivation to work hard to find it. While the availability of palatable foods – rich in sugar and fat – are commonplace these days, our hunger signals have not changed much since then. In the body, highly palatable foods work especially well for weakening satiety signals and activating hunger signals [14]. During our evolution, this was useful, as palatable foods were rare but important sources of energy, and overeating them when they were available contributed to our survival. The problem now is that we live in an era of plenty where finding palatable food is no longer a challenge – on the contrary, the challenge is now how to avoid them!

Built-in food preferences

As food has become more and more available almost everywhere, it isn't easy to avoid eating what we are designed to enjoy the most: sugar, fat and salt. From birth, we are programmed to prefer these tastes – and to avoid tastes like bitter and sour. As is extensively explained in the brilliant book *The end of overeating* by David A. Kessler, our brains are wired to like certain nutrients more than other. "We are designed to crave foods rich in fat, sugar and salt, preferably all mixed together to form an irresistible combination that arouses our brains and activates our built-in reward systems". Even newborns and young children are wired to prefer sweet and salty over bitter flavors [15, 16]. This matters, as adults who eat more sweets are also prone to eat more fruits (but not vegetables) [17] – again showing how our built-in taste preferences can affect our eating habits.

Without the limitations to our food supply seen in history, it is easy to see how we can lose control of our eating. And we have. Just look at the high number of overweight and obese individuals in most countries nowadays – people who I am sure would prefer to be slim and healthy.

Food as comfort

Ah emotions...what would life be like without emotions? It is very hard to imagine, but a good guess is that we would probably be like those robots in science fiction movies. But what do emotions have to do with food? Everything! Emotions are commonly defined as a mental state that occurs spontaneously, often followed by changes to the body. Emotions can influence your eating behavior very much. Some people eat when they are angry, others when they are bored. Still others overeat when depressed or happy. Considering that we are all different, it is very difficult to generalize as to which emotion has the greatest effect on eating, and it probably also differs depending on where you are and your emotional state [18]. The food you eat, its type, amount and the frequency all depend on many factors, but definitely do not always reflect your nutritional needs.

In special cases, the relationship with food may even become abnormal. Emotional eating is diagnosed when strong emotions are often present at meals, or when eating occurs regularly without hunger. Even for people with a normal relationship to food, eating to make you feel better is a telltale sign. Emotional eating episodes can occur sporadically (such as when something happens to make you feel extra low) or on a regular basis, and more often than not take place in secret using foods rich in sugar and fat. And more, emotional eating is more common when people are alone, more likely to occur at dinner or snack time than at breakfast, and often happens in combination with meals eaten at home rather than when eating out [19]. Perhaps most importantly, emotional eating does not discriminate by social class, skin color or sex. It is, however, more common in overweight and obese people – as well as amongst frequent dieters [20].

Like most of us, you are probably susceptible to your emotions every now and then – and sometimes, despite your best efforts, you will use food to modify bad feelings. Successful Losers are also affected by such behavior. However, they do not let their emotions control them for long. Instead, they find constructive ways to deal with their feelings. In a moment of anger, instead of releasing their frustration with a box of chocolate, they go to the gym or for a walk. Their secret is to learn to tell emotional eating from hunger even in the heat of the moment, and to develop other strategies to deal with strong emotions when they happen.

The high price of convenience

With today's hectic lifestyles, you may feel that you do not have time to do anything anymore. In my life, there are millions of things that I just have to do – while free time in which to do them is a luxury. Unfortunately, as a society, we have adopted a compromise that gives a low priority to such essential things as food. More often than not, many of us now end up choosing our meals for convenience rather than nutritional value. We buy ready-made frozen foods, go to fast-food restaurants and order takeout on a regular basis. No wonder then that we have been labeled the fast-food nation! That might not have been a bad thing if all of the so-called "convenience food" was not so unhealthy, affordable and, well, fast. The typical frozen dish or take-out meal contains cheap but harmful saturated and trans fats, huge amounts of sodium (which contributes to a high blood pressure), artificial preservatives, sweet but caloric corn syrup and more.

And our fast-food is cheap! Price – not only in dollars and cents, but also in time saved – goes hand in hand with convenience. How often do you compare foods by their price tag? And how often do you actually compare how healthy they are? Many people are knowledgeable about healthy food choices, but when confronted with the usual trade-off between price and nutritional value, they usually choose the cheaper food [21]. This is true to such an extent that the price of healthy food is perceived as one of the key barriers to healthier eating by the majority of consumers.

In order to test how much the price of foods influences consumer choices, a team of scientists lead by Dr. Simone A. French from the University of Minnesota studied the effect of price reductions for low-fat snacks in vending machines at work sites and secondary schools. All the vending machines at each site had both healthy and unhealthy snacks, with the prices of the healthy snacks reduced relative to the unhealthy snacks by 10%, 25% and 50%. Not surprisingly, when prices were lowered, the sales of healthy snacks increased dramatically. And more, the greater the reduction in price the more healthy snacks were sold – both at work places and schools [22]! Even small price differences have large effects on purchase decisions! So, price really does matter! That is why you and I should both make it a habit to consciously compare the long-term benefits of paying more for a healthier food. Just think of how much you will save on insurance co-payments if you are fit and healthy!

Habit is stronger than nature

We are creatures of habit! We like what is familiar to us, and most of us do not wake up every day and invent a whole new breakfast menu. Instead, we are likely to stick with what we are used to. Unless you make a conscious effort to change and improve your diet, it will not happen.

As we have seen, our food preferences are partly dictated by evolutionary programming, but they can be changed by repetitive exposure to new foods. For example, children who are exposed to a varied diet become more open to trying new foods. These children simply get used to trying new things, and the more new foods they try, the easier it becomes for them to adopt a varied and healthy diet [23]. And if small children can get used to eating new foods, I bet that you can too! Believe me, healthy eating is a learned behavior that anyone can master! That said, it takes time to adapt to a healthier diet – so persist in trying new foods that are healthy (but not yet part of your daily diet) and you will eventually end up liking them. Just ask any Successful Loser!

Peer pressure matters

We are social beings and that is no secret! We like to belong to a group and to feel as a part of society. If you are like most people, you like to do what others are doing – not standing out by being contrary all the time. This is also true when it comes to your eating habits.

When researchers decided to investigate how peer pressure influences children's eating habits, they found that using videos of other children of a similar age happily eating foods that had previously been rejected by the children in the study, they could increase the participating children's acceptance of these foods. And not only of a specific food, but of whole groups of food such as fruit and vegetables. So now you know what cartoons to show your fussy child – those that feature happy young animals munching on leafy greens and fruit! Obviously, this type of study is harder to perform with grown-ups. However, doctors at Harvard Medical School have found that people who have friends, siblings or spouses that are overweight themselves have a greater risk of becoming fat [24]. To me, this implies that the social norms that we share with our social circle have an important impact on our waistline also as adults.

Now that you know the main reasons why you eat what you eat, you would think it should be easier to make healthier and smarter food choices. But there are powerful forces conspiring against you living a healthy lifestyle. Does this mean that you are destined to be fat? Read the next chapter to find out!

Chapter 2 in a nutshell

❖ Food is what nourishes and sustains our bodies, but it is also used to modify our emotions. Emotional eating is far too common and if not addressed it can ruin your chances of becoming a Successful Loser.

❖ Our food choices are influenced by our biological programming. We are designed to enjoy foods rich in sugar, salt and fat – and we certainly do!

❖ Convenience and price influence our food choices more than we think. So, make a conscious decision to choose your foodstuffs based on their nutritional value – it will be cheaper in the long run!

❖ Most of us are creatures of habit and eat what we are used to eating. Successful Losers are no exception

– that's why they make sure to consciously practice healthy eating until it becomes their new normal.

❖ As social beings we are strongly influenced by the eating habits of those close to us.

[3]

Are you destined to be fat?

Our bodies are designed to hang on to every calorie that we eat presumably this ability was a great survival advantage in ancient times, when finding enough food was difficult. With industrialization, the production, availability, distribution and consumption of food changed practically overnight but our bodies did not. And the human body's inability to adapt to this situation of always available and plentiful foods has resulted in an epidemic of obesity in the United States and most of the world. While it may seem unfair today, our bodies were simply never prepared for this age of 24 hours-open supermarkets and fast-food restaurants.

Obesity epidemic

Over the last decades, overweight and obesity has reached epidemic proportions in most, if not all, parts of the world! Worldwide, excess body-weight affects 1.5 billion adults – leading some to call it *globesity*. In the United States, one out of every two Americans is overweight or obese [25]. In 2010, no American state had less than 20% prevalence of obesity. Thirty-six states had a prevalence of 25% or more; in 12 of these 30% or more of the citizens were obese – one person out of every three! [26]. Even scarier, by 2015 the World Health Organization predicts that globally, 2.3 billion people will be overweight and 700 million will be obese [27].

If the obesity epidemic does not end – or worse, continue to escalate, there will be severe consequences not only at the individual level, but also for societies as a whole. A group of scientists from Johns Hopkins School of Public Health, predicts that should nothing change by 2030, 86% of adult Americans will be overweight or obese. By 2048, all American adults will be overweight or obese, causing the health-care costs related to obesity and overweight to double every decade until then. This means that already in 2030 1/5th of all healthcare spending – $957 billion [28]! – will go to treating the consequences of overweight and obesity. Put another way, every American would on average pay $3.000 US dollars per year for treating preventable obesity related diseases – can you think of a better way to spend that money? These are scary numbers, but things do not have to turn out so badly. The time for change has come – and there has never been so much knowledge and so many treatments available to help you lose weight; however, you must first make up your mind and decide to become a Successful Loser!

Why is bad to be fat?

The health risks linked to overweight and obesity are real and serious. When it gets to the point where you have been diagnosed with obesity, it is no longer a matter of how good or bad you look – but rather how you will survive to a ripe old age! Obesity is a serious health condition that has been proven to lead to most of the big killer diseases of industrialized societies. To motivate you, here are some scary facts about the most common diseases linked to overweight and obesity.

Heart disease and high blood cholesterol

Increased production of "bad" (or LDL) cholesterol almost always occurs with obesity – along with a reduced ability to deal with sugar taken up in the gut. There are 71 million Americans with elevated cholesterol levels, but only 34 million of them receive treatment [29]. Unfortunately, most of those treated receive expensive medications rather than help to change their lifestyle – a scientifically proven, better choice! Although the resulting control of cholesterol is improving, it still remains low [29]. High levels of "bad" cholesterol is linked to an increased risk of developing cardiovascular disease (also known as heart disease), and heart disease is the number one killer in the United States – more than one million people suffer heart attacks per year! It is clear that obesity caused by overeating is the major factor behind increased cholesterol levels, and it is also the most important risk factor for cardiovascular disease along with smoking.

Diabetes mellitus

Diabetes mellitus type 2 (or adult onset diabetes) is the visible tip of a very large iceberg of metabolic disease linked to overweight. In fact, today more than 25 million Americans have type 2 diabetes, and as a result they are at increased risk of cardiovascular diseases, stroke and an early death. Adult onset diabetes occurs as a consequence of obesity in most people that develop the disease. And in those that already suffer from type 2 diabetes, weight loss and a more active lifestyle can mean the difference between a relatively normal life and daily insulin injections [30]. Keep in mind that even middling amounts of fat around the waistline can lead to insulin resistance and sugar intolerance – which may rapidly progress to full-blown diabetes. Weight loss, a healthy diet, and regular physical activity are some of the best preventative actions to take [31].

High blood pressure

Hypertension is a fancy way of saying high blood pressure. The majority of hypertensive individuals have only a mildly elevated blood pressure. But even a 10% elevation in blood pressure from normal (say 130/90 instead of 120/80 mmHg) is associated with increased risk of heart disease, kidney disease and premature death. Our unhealthy diets also contribute to hypertension. High-fat fast-food, for example, is commonly also rich in salt to make it taste better! Eating too much salt (even if you are not aware of it!)

can increase your blood pressure to harmful levels by forcing your heart to pump extra water soaked up by all the salt in the circulation. The best way to prevent or treat high blood pressure is through a healthy diet and regular exercise. In fact, many people with mild obesity-associated hypertension will normalize their blood pressure as soon as they lose any significant amount of weight (5-10% of their current weight). However, once you stop exercising or gain your weight back, your blood pressure goes up again. So maintaining a healthy weight is essential if you want to keep your blood pressure under control.

Cancers

Being overweight or obese can dramatically increase your chance of developing cancer, and it also makes it more difficult to treat cancer once you have developed the disease. Indeed, The American Cancer Society has linked obesity to the rising incidence of many common cancers, including breast, ovarian, colon, uterine, prostate, pancreatic, gallbladder, and kidney cancers [32]. Also, when an individual moves from a country with healthier eating habits to the United States, hers or his risk of breast or prostate cancer increases dramatically within one generation. I am not saying all common cancers are caused by overweight or that all overweight people develop cancer. What I am saying is that staying or becoming slim and healthy really makes sense.

Psychosocial problems

While many physical effects of overweight and obesity are easy to measure, there are also important psychological consequences of being overweight. They include sexual dysfunction, worse job performance, a lower social status and less self-esteem – all of which obviously lead to a worse quality of life! Indeed, according to a regularly performed national health survey [33], obesity related health issues have drastically decreased Americans' quality of life during the past 15 years. As you know, being fat is both traumatic and one of the best ways to shorten your life. If that does not motivate you to act now and become a Successful Loser, I do not know what will!

Our "fat" environment

Sometimes, despite your best efforts to eat healthier or exercise more, it seems like the whole world conspires to make you eat poorly and be physically inactive. Just think about all those food advertised on TV and how easy, tasty and cheap they are – only one phone call away! Even the best intentions and the hardest resolve can quickly dissipate when facing such discouraging circumstances. That is what we call an obesogenic environment, meaning a setting which promotes consumption of a high calorie, high sugar diet of tasty and cheap foods, while minimizing as much as possible the amount of physical activity required in daily life [34]. For example, the rapid spread of vending machines in convenient locations, home delivery of junk-food, and the relative lack of bike lanes compared to highways are all part of our obesogenic environment. Our days as hunter-gatherers are long gone, and have been replaced by sedentary days in front of a screen together with enormous quantities of junk food. Only during the last 30 years, the total daily calorie intake of the average American has increased from 2400 to 2600 kcal for men and from 1500 to 1900 kcal for women [35]. Meanwhile, the amount of calories used during physical activity decreased in both men and women.

It is not surprising then that our obesogenic environment has been suggested as the major cause of the obesity epidemic. For most of us, it is almost impossible to keep a healthy weight when tempted with so many unhealthy options! All tailored to appeal to our primitive survival instincts – encouraging overeating (e.g., large portion sizes; increased availability of cheap tasty, energy-dense foods and snacks; increased marketing of sweetened beverages, etc.) and discouraging physical activity (e.g., television, computer and internet use; sedentary occupations and cars).

Prominent experts have suggested that to win the fight against obesity we may be forced to make drastic changes to our environment [36]. But while you may not be in a position to change society and save its many members destined to die young from obesity related health issues, you can save yourself by changing your response to the obesogenic world of the present. Successful Losers do just that – and manage to stay fit even in the most tempting of circumstances! Despite the obesogenic environment, they manage to introduce and maintain healthy lifestyle habits! But, which are these healthy lifestyle habits? Keep on reading and you will find out. Later on in this book you will discover how Successful Losers handle their personal environment to maximize their successes!

Your set point: breed or bread?

Being overweight is the consequence of a complicated relationship between genetics and environment. Through evolution, we have developed a finely tuned system to maintain body weight within a relatively narrow range despite a large daily variability in energy intake and expenditure. Indeed, you and everyone else come with a weight equilibrium "set point". This point is set so that your body is well-equipped to protect you against weight loss during caloric deprivation enabling you to survive periods when little food was available. Unfortunately, nothing in our past has prepared us to live in a land of plenty such as today [37]. A classical example of this is the study [38] of 12 pairs of identical twins (same genes) showing the effects of genetics on weight gain or weight loss in response to a high calorie diet. For a period of 100 days, all the twins were given an extra 1000 kcal per day on top of what was needed for weight maintenance. At the end of the study, there were more differences in weight gain, muscle mass and fat mass between than within the pairs. At 18 months after the end of the study, all of the pairs had reduced to roughly their initial weight. Unfortunately for some of us, the science behind the study concluded that when the environment is controlled to be the same, the decisive factor determining weight gain or weight loss is genetic [38, 39].

So, life really is not fair! Some of us are indeed more prone to be fat than others – and that is a fact! But your genetic predisposition does not determine your waistline! It is true that there are differences in metabolism, which can make some individuals more efficient at burning calories than others. Still, by far the most common reasons for differences in the tendency to gain or lose weight relate to lifestyle and habits. Thus, while you may have genes that make you prone to be overweight, this extra weight only appears when you let it. Yours, mine, and everybody else's body fat is the result of a very simple math: if you consistently take in more calories than you burn, you are going to gain weight regardless of your genetic make-up.

"Your genetic predisposition does not determine your waistline"

Indeed, most "normal" people are genetically vulnerable to obesity when consuming a high calorie diet. And the growing proportion of obese Americans indicates that the majority of us are now doing just that! Physical activity is also important in our calorie-rich society that the amount of time that you spend watching television every day is now able to tell me how fat you are [11, 40]! So, anyone can figure out that if you move less but eat the same, you will gain weight. Likewise, if you eat the same but move more, you will lose weight. Now, the question is what you are going to do about it? Start by no longer blaming your parents or genes for your love handles – then take control of your life and achieve your goals!

How do you know if you are fat?

While being fat is a descriptive term based on prejudice and appearance, overweight and obesity are labels for ranges of weight that are greater than what is generally considered healthy. Commonly, obesity is diagnosed by using the body mass index, also known as BMI. BMI is calculated by dividing one's body weight (lbs) by the square of one's height (ft) multiplied by 703. If your BMI is below 18.5, you are considered underweight (which is also not healthy), if it is 18.5-24.9 you have a healthy weight, while BMI from 25 to 29.9 means that you are overweight, 30-39.9 is considered obese (clinical obesity) and above 40 is classified as morbidly obese (and very dangerous). BMI is by no means a perfect tool, but it is the most widely used method because for most people it correlates well with the amount of body fat. However, in some cases BMI can falsely indicate that someone is obese when in reality he or she is not. For example, a bodybuilder probably has a BMI indicating overweight or obesity, but in reality has a lot of extra weight from muscles not fat – of which there may be very little! However, if you are not a bodybuilder, a professional athlete, or suffer from certain diseases that alter your body composition you can safely use BMI to find out if you have the right weight for your height.

Body Mass Index	**Classification**
Below 18.5	Underweight
18.5 to 24.9	Healthy weight
25.0 to 29.9	Overweight
30 or 39.9	Obese
40 or higher	Morbidly obese

Another easy and effective way to find out if your health is at risk because of obesity is to measure your waist circumference. A waist circumference above 40 inches (or 102 cm) for men and above 35 inches (88 cm) for women is a sign of excess fat [41]. This abdominal fat also contains higher amounts of metabolically active fat that is easily transported to your liver, where it is turned into cholesterol and released into your bloodstream – contributing to the formation of plaques in the artery walls. That's why you are more likely to have a high cholesterol, high blood pressure, and cardiovascular disease when you have excess abdominal fat.

In fact, waist circumference is a better indicator of complications of obesity than BMI, especially among certain populations. For example, elderly people with less muscle mass tend to have BMI values that underestimate their risk, while physically active people with a lot of muscle get a falsely elevated risk by using BMI. In these and other cases, it may be better to measure your waist circumference. Use a tape measure to measure your waist circumference all the way around just at the top of your (hopefully easily located!) hip bone, making sure to hold the measure straight like a belt and tightly in place over a bare abdomen. Make sure that you are not holding your breath (however tempting!) then read the measurement.

Gender	Reference values	Health risks
Woman	35 inches (88 cm) or more	Sleep apnea, type 2 diabetes, heart disease, cancer, high
Man	40 inches (102 cm) or more	blood pressure and psychosocial problems

If you are one of the many people with a waist circumference above the safe values, you are not alone! In the United States, it is estimated that nearly two thirds (68%) of adults are above these values and are consequently at risk of developing diseases related to obesity. The good news is that is never too late to change your lifestyle and start losing weight – even small changes can yield great results. But the 1 million dollar question is: Are you ready to become a Successful Loser?

Chapter 3 in a nutshell

- ❖ The obesity epidemic has a very high cost both at a societal and personal level. Not only does it cost us billions as a society, but it also costs many people their lives – and it could cost yours if you let it!
- ❖ There are strong obesogenic forces working to make you fat. So, if you want to be a Successful Loser you have to find ways around them that work for you.
- ❖ Yes, some people have genes that make it easier for them to stay slim, but if you don't belong to this category you can still be slim; you just have to work harder!
- ❖ By using BMI, you can easily find out if you are in a healthy weight range or not.

Another way of measuring if your health is at risk due to overweight is by measuring and keeping track of your waist circumference.

[4]

Are you ready to become a Successful Loser?

Why do people change? That's in fact a difficult and very interesting question! Most of us would like to change something, and you probably know someone (maybe yourself?) who is always complaining about some aspect of life. I know someone very close to me (don't tell my mother that I am telling you this!) who is always complaining that she is too fat and should lose weight – but year after year complain is all she does, while her weight remains the same. By all means, my mother is a very accomplished person who has succeeded in many aspects of life – but when it comes to her weight she is in a never ending battle with the scales. In this chapter I will guide you through a journey to discover if you really are ready to tackle your weight – and if you are not, how to get there. Always remember though, that I am not able to make decisions for you. You are the only one who can decide what to do. All that I can do is point to the right path and give you the tools to empower you to get the best from your body.

Before you can get anywhere near your dream body, you need to turn off the auto-pilot. You have got to realize and truly believe that change is possible and that it is not as hard as you might think. A full commitment held for longer than just a few days is all it takes to start creating changes that others may call miracles. Before trying to change anything, including your habits, you have to find out how motivated you are. In this chapter I describe commonly agreed stages on the way to achieving change. Usually people fit into one or more of the stages of change. After reading the description, you may realize that you are not yet motivated enough to change at all. That is ok, and you can use the scientifically proven techniques later on this book to help you motivate yourself. After all, you must be at least a little bit motivated – or else you would not be reading this book!

Stages of change

Stages of change is a model designed to explain the process people go through before they change a bad habit – be it overeating, a sedentary lifestyle, binge drinking or smoking. The model is based on a lot of interesting research showing that people who successfully change their behavior go through a series of five stages of readiness - usually cycling through them three to four times before really changing a behavior [42]. I believe that it is critically important to recognize where you are in the stages of change model, so that you can set appropriate goals and take the right action. According to the expert in self-change who developed the model [42], each stage requires a different strategy to pass. If you set goals that you are not yet ready to fulfill, you are sure to fail and get discouraged. Similarly, if you choose goals that you have already mastered, you will delay your progress and may even delude yourself that you are already there. By matching your goals to your stage of change, you will maximize your ability to effect change. For more detailed information about the science behind this model of behavioral changing, I recommend that you read the brilliant book *Changing for Good* by James O. Prochaska, John C. Norcross and Carlo C. Diclement.

Stage 1: Pre-contemplation – you don't yet see why you would need to change

Pre-contemplators resist change – even thinking about change! While they may temporarily modify their behavior if there is enough external pressure, once the pressure is removed they rapidly go back to their old ways. Pre-contemplators are often discouraged by earlier failed attempts and do not want to think about their problem, because they feel that the situation (or even themselves) is hopeless [42].

During this stage, you lack deep knowledge of your problem while inertia prevents you from even considering changing your life. Maybe you are not even conscious of the consequences of your actions. It is very likely that, even though you are not very happy as you are, your life seems more comfortable than having to contemplate changing your behavior. If you are at this stage of change, you might have experienced your family members or friends suggesting that you should lose weight or start going to the gym – but you think that you do not need to lose weight and the only reason you are overweight is because you have a large bone structure. Or you have tried every diet on Earth and are convinced that you are a complete failure or somehow different from everyone else.

Stage 2: Contemplation – you know it is important to change, but...

This stage is also known as the "I'll do it when..." phase. At this point, you acknowledge that you have a problem and start to consider various ways to solve it. For example, you may now know the health risks of being overweight and are aware that fat prevents you from living a full life. But you still do not make weight loss a priority in your life, instead justifying your overweight by blaming exterior circumstances such as lack of time, money, opportunities or ability.

Indeed, while people at this stage may have vague plans to change, they are often not ready to take action yet. In fact, most people remain in the contemplation stage for years. You might be in this stage of change if you constantly keep finding excuses to justify your inaction: "I will stop buying take-out food for dinner when I have more time to cook healthy home-cooked meals" or "I can't exercise because I cannot afford to pay for an expensive gym membership". Does it sound familiar? Is that where you are?

Stage 3: Preparation – you want to change, but how?

In the preparation stage, you are planning to make changes in the near future and you feel so sure about this that you are willing to announce the coming change to those close to you. However, secretly you still doubt if you are able and willing to do what it takes to really make the change. If you are in this phase, you are not only aware of the importance of losing weight, but you are also informed and concerned about what might happen if you don't change. In fact, you may already have taken steps to achieve your goals – you just have not been able to follow through. You might have enrolled in a gym but never go there, planned to eat more healthily by going to the sushi bar at work but been lured by your colleagues to the usual pizza place, or bought and read some healthy cook books but never actually made any recipes. Fortunately, at this stage you recognize that you are the one responsible for changing your life – but unfortunately daily obligations have so far kept you from making a long-term effort. Being where you are, you should know that this trial and error preparation stage is necessary. Those who cut the time spent in preparation short lower their chances of success later.

In this stage, it is important to develop a realistic, detailed plan of action to carry you through to success – tailored to your life by you, the expert. If you are at this stage, you have made firm commitment to change, and are working on the how rather than the why or when. You know yourself and your body well enough to realize that if you cook all your weekly dinner meals on Sunday evenings and freeze them in small portions, you will be able to have a home-cooked dinner every night instead of take-out. You also realize that you do not need a fancy gym membership to exercise as you hate to be looked at by other people – instead you set up your living room as your own personal gym and walk to and from work most days of the week.

Stage 4: Action – you will now do whatever it takes to become a Successful Loser!

The action stage is the busiest stage in the process of change – and it therefore also requires the most dedication and stamina. You are now putting your previously made plans into action. This stage is when you actually start going regularly to the gym, cooking healthy meals, and refusing to buy potato chips. You know that life will not always be easy on you, you also know that there will be inevitable setbacks and problems, but you also know that only by deciding to do whatever it takes to achieve your goals will you succeed!

"Lasting change only occurs when you are ready,
informed and 100% committed to a new, healthy lifestyle"

While the action stage usually receives the most attention, it is worthless without the knowledge, planning and dedication that you have built up during your passage through the other stages! The action stage is therefore not the only one that you should consider as progress towards achieving your goals. Be proud of yourself even if you fail at your first attempts at action – remember all of the other stages that you have gone through and keep your eyes on the prize! If you are at this stage – the name says it all – you are putting the plans you made during the preparation stage into action! You have taken an important step towards achieving your goals – now all you need is the willpower to keep going regardless! You are now a Successful Loser in the making!

Stage 5: Maintenance – keeping up the good work!

Contrary to what you may expect, the action stage is not the final stage in the change process. The maintenance stage comes after, and it is where you consolidate your gains from the action stage and work to prevent relapses. We have all managed to change a bad habit only for it to come right back! We all know someone who lost many pounds on a diet, but then regained them all a few months later. You might have lost weight, but now is the time to work to maintain your sexy new body!

The maintenance stage is actually life-long, always ongoing, and critically important. You are in the maintenance stage when you go to the gym even if you come home from work tired, or if you order salad in a restaurant even when everyone else is eating pizza and making fun of you. The maintenance stage may sound even worse than your current life, but it isn't! Having changed, your new you is the new normal – and you will for the most part automatically do what you before fought so hard to achieve. In fact, you can now afford to cut yourself some slack once in a while – you are only human after all! However, this stage requires constant vigilance to prevent you from slipping back to your old ways – even after years or decades.

As I said, in the maintenance stage healthy habits become just that – habits that effortlessly form part of your routine. You now belong to the small elite who have lost their excess weight for good; you are now a Successful Loser and can set an example for others. You not only know – but actually experience – that lasting change only occurs when you are ready, informed and 100% committed to a new, healthy lifestyle [7]. This is what distinguishes Successful Losers from all others!

In the stage of change theory developed by Dr. Prochaska and colleagues there is yet another stage – termination. In this stage, the struggle with unhealthy habits is over and such behaviors will never again return (the authors give the example of giving up smoking). However, I and many other experts do not believe that change involving certain other problems can ever reach the termination stage. I would rate eating habits and exercise routines amongst them. These behaviors are simply so rooted in our brains that no amount of change can get them out – and with good reason (imagine if you lost the will to eat or the desire to rest)! Unfortunately, that means that you will never reach the termination stage for most of the lifestyle habits that you adopt after reading this book. Rather, you should expect to continue in the maintenance phase. However, as demonstrated by the Successful Losers, this simply means that you will have to work to keep your healthy habits – also after many years of healthy living.

What's in it for you?

Every aspect of our lives contains good and bad – and these change over time, so that, meaning that what is good in the short-term (eating a candy bar) may be bad in the long-term (because you may gain weight and get diabetes). However as hard as it may be to believe, even the worst habits offer some gain – or we would not engage in them! "Bad habits" may help us to avoid discomfort, stay in touch with cherished friends, belong to a certain group, save us money or simply just give us a buzz. However, you also always have to pay a price for clinging to "bad habits" – which is why they are "bad". When it comes to overeating and overweight, this price might be deteriorating health, an unsatisfying social or love life, a feeling of missing out on something, a lack of energy or even discrimination at work or in society. Take a moment to consider the bad habits you have and list the pros and cons of each – a balance sheet of your habits, so to speak. Are you willing and able to pay the price? Now, consider how you plan to change your life and list the benefits and costs of giving up your current habits and for each new "good habit" that you realistically expect to adopt. Does this new cost seem worth the effort? For example, what is a longer life or a higher self-esteem worth to you? You are the only one who knows.

When you are done, you should have a pretty clear idea of what benefits you get from your current lifestyle, and if the new life you are contemplating is worth the hassle of change to you. If you decide that it is not (be honest to yourself!), you are simply not ready for change yet! Instead of trying and failing to adopt a completely new lifestyle, go back and look at the facts again. Learn about all the negative health consequences of being overweight – and of all of the benefits derived from eating well and using your body as it was intended to be used. Remember, only when you truly feel ready to change is it worth to start planning that change in detail.

Having decided to be a Successful Loser once and for all, you need to tailor your own strategies to achieve your goals. In fact, the best expert on you is yourself. In the next chapter, you will discover how to set goals that are realistic and attainable.

Chapter 4 in a nutshell

❖ To become a Successful Loser, you need to be fully committed to change your unhealthy lifestyle into a new, healthy one.

❖ Before you truly change anything in your life, you will need to go through a series of predictable stages – and it is impossible to skip one stage and go directly to your new life.

❖ In the pre-contemplation stage, you won't even realize that you have a problem – and therefore you will be unwilling to consider changing anything about the way you live.

❖ During the contemplation phase, you become intellectually aware that you would like to change some things in your life, but you are not emotionally and personally motivated enough to make any serious attempt at change beyond gathering information (such as buying this book!).

❖ In the preparation stage, you become convinced that change is necessary and you start to plan how to achieve the results that you want. Rushing this stage by adopting somebody else's solution (for example a miracle diet) is a common mistake!

❖ Following preparation comes the action phase, where you put your plans for change into action. This is where most people fail, usually because they lack enough self-knowledge or attempt too drastic changes all at once.

❖ The maintenance stage comes last in the change process – but lasts the longest! It starts the moment you have successfully changed your life. Succeeding here means to keep on practicing the healthy habits that made you a Successful Loser in the first place!

❖ To get started with changing your life, make a list of all of the things that you like about your current "bad" (unhealthy) habits. Then, make a new of all the benefits you would get if you adopted "good" (healthy) habits. Is it worth it?

[5]

Don't bite off more than you can chew – setting realistic goals

Congratulations! You have finally decided to become a Successful Loser. From now on, you are only going to eat healthy foods in small portions, abstain from alcohol, kiss sweets goodbye, hit the gym 5 times a week, cycle to work every day, take your dog/kids to play outside more often, limit your TV time to one hour per day, lose half of your body weight in six months and keep up this lifestyle for the rest of your life. Simple? Of course not – impossible is more like it! Unlike so many of the magician dietitians out there with their miracle diets, I don't think that it is realistic to change your life in 10, 30 or even 60 days – let alone change it completely! Do you want to know the main reason why so many people with good intentions fail to lose weight? Because they set unrealistic goals, fail to reach them and give up trying for fear of feeling even more like a failure than they already do! If you are overweight now, it did not happen overnight – it took you years to pile on all the extra weight. But when it comes to losing weight, most people seem to think becoming slim happens at the drop of a hat – or at least over 10 frenetic days of eating nothing but liquids! Of course, deep down they know as well as you that the diet is more to lose their bad consciences than to lose weight, and that having suffered for a short while means that they can safely go back to their ways for another year!

*"Goals are guides that help you get from where you are
to where you want to be!"*

Like everyone else, you also know that to achieve your goals, you have to both make them realistic and work hard; otherwise, you are only setting yourself up for failure – a major killer of self-confidence and change initiative. By now, having made up your mind to change and formulated a long-term goal – to lose one hundred pounds and keep it off, to be so physically active that you can run (and finish!) a marathon, to eat so healthily that you can get off your diabetes drugs, or something else. The next step in your strategy to bring forth change should be to break down your big goal into many smaller and realistic ones to be achieved one by one over time.

You will learn how you can do this soon, but for now you will have to take my word for it that this type of goal-setting is an effective strategy for long-term changes in dietary and physical activity habits [43]. It also works well for the management of chronic diseases – such as diabetes and high blood pressure – where your health depends largely on how well you follow a prescribed diet, physical activity, and/or medication [44, 45].

Goal setting is an effective and widely used tool in fields from sports to the corporate world. Goals are guides that help you get from where you are to where you want to be! Think of them as way end-points – not your final destination.

Timing is everything!

We are in a constant struggle between our short-term and long-term needs and wants (we'll get back to this). Goals are no exception! As expected, goals and deadlines in the short term are easier to focus on, simply because they are closer in time. But achieving short-term goals can motivate you to take further action; making small changes one after the other provides you with successes on which to build [46]. On the other hand, long-term goals are often what you really want to attain – but unless you are of an impressively patient and focused nature, chances are that a goal so far into the future does not provide you with enough motivation or indication of progress, increasing the risk that you will delay starting or completely abandon your task before it is finished.

Rome was not built in one day!

If you are like most people, when you want something you want it as soon as possible. Not surprisingly, research into the setting and achievement of goals shows that individuals who set specific, short-term goals incrementally leading up to their long-term desire have a much greater chance of success than do those who immediately try for their long-term goal [47]. So don't be hasty! A realistic plan contains several short-term goals (e.g. drink 8 glasses of water daily, eat leafy greens with every meal, or have [a healthy] breakfast every day) that ultimately lead you to achieve your desired goal (e.g. to lose 30 pounds in six months).

For those of us who have a lot of weight to lose, it may be daunting to even imagine the large amount of change needed to achieve a healthy weight. Don't despair! Even a very modest weight loss (5% of body weight) or a small increase in daily physical activity (10 minutes of walking 3 times a day) produces major health benefits. A small weight loss can improve not only one disease, but a whole spectrum (everything from heart disease to sexual dysfunction to diabetes and back pain) [48, 49]. Also remember that maintaining a modest weight loss is much more beneficial than losing a larger amount of weight and gaining it back.

By breaking down the process and creating several smaller goals that may be attained relatively quickly, you will encourage yourself and create easily observed and celebrated successes that will eventually lead to your bigger goal! In fact, this approach has been proven by science, and Successful Losers everywhere [50]!

You really are unique

How you pursue your goals is influenced by how and when you set that goal to begin with. Simply put, goals that you decided on yourself are much easier to attain [51]. Performance and persistence are just more likely to occur when goals and strategies come from within than as a result of external forces (think nagging spouse or picky diet buddy). Assigned goals are a form of external manipulation which many of us instinctively resist [52]. Successful Losers know that to achieve any goal, the motivation and the game plan must come from within. They always set their own realistic but challenging goals instead of allowing others to do it for them. As a result, they attain what we all dream about – one small step at a time.

Do not compare yourself to others!

We all know about someone who lost an incredible amount of weight in a short time and became a triathlon athlete, or who was a couch potato but now goes to the gym seven days a week, or someone who cooks healthy home-made meals every day despite having a full-time job and four kids. These are the people who effortlessly seem to make life look like a walk in the park – maybe you are one of these people, but most of us are not!

We compare ourselves to others more than we would like to admit. We are social animals after all, preferring to belong to a group and be liked by everyone. And there is nothing wrong with this – in fact it is natural. But it can cause you a lot of unnecessary distress if you compare yourself with a whole electronic universe of others (some of them not real), or with only the sides of others that they wish to show you. The risk is that you adopt the goals and ideals of these others as you own. Remember, you are unique, and you work and feel best when your life is run according to your rules and wishes – not those of others!

Be specific

How specific a goal is plays an important part in determining your motivation for achieving it, as well as how detailed and therefore workable your strategies for success will be. Specific goals, such as going to the gym 3 days a week for one month, or eating 5 portions of fruits and vegetables per day, are more effective and lead to higher levels of success than general goals such as being more physically active or eating more healthily. Besides that, general goals work poorly because they do not allow you to verify that you are progressing [53]. Instead, use easy to measure (think numbers!) targets and display your progress on your very own "scoreboard". You may keep it to yourself if you wish, but goals that are openly declared are helpful because they reduce the risk of "target drift", which means that you consciously or subconsciously modify your goal over time in order to make it easier to attain [46, 53]. When setting goals, Successful Losers have a clear picture of what they want to achieve, how and when.

I suggest that you do the same, start by setting easily measured, short-term goals. For example, let's assume your goal is to be physically active for five hours a week. Take a paper, stick it on the wall next to the TV and write down when you start and stop watching TV every day for a week. Using this information, work out a schedule that cuts the time you spend watching TV in half. Aim for at least five hours cut, and instead spend those hours walking briskly around your block while listening to music that you like (or a podcast) instead. Each time that you get home after a walk, put a large cross on the paper and reward yourself in some (non-caloric) way!

Now it is your turn to come up with a smart and easy way to achieve your personal short-term goals. The more specific your goals are, the more likely you are to find a working strategy, stick to it – and succeed! Please take a few minutes to think about and write down what your specific short-term and long-term goals are – and which strategies and actions you can take today in order to attain them – as well as when they will be attained.

Keep your eyes on the prize!

As you start achieving your short-term goals, you can start challenging yourself by setting more difficult and longer-term goals – remember, if a task does not cause you to cringe, it is because you have already mastered it and it is time to move on to new challenges!

To do that, it helps to consider your reward system. What motivates you to pursue your goals? Is it the feeling of accomplishment and pride, an improved health, to fit in your old clothes, the admiration of your peers or the sensation that you are living your life to the fullest? Motivation comes in many shape and forms! Often, it is disguised as love, fear, anger, pride, fulfillment or expectation. Positive as well as negative motivation can both be helpful if used correctly (think, if I do not go to the gym tonight, I will not have my usual glass of wine this Saturday).

As we have seen, the most important thing with motivation seems to be that it comes from inside – but that also means that it is credible to you! It is no use threatening yourself with consequences if you know already today that you will not follow through with the punishment! We are all different people who value different things in life. By finding what it is that drives you, you will be able to strategically use this knowledge to motivate you to achieve your goals. But remember, you are trying to change your life to improve its quality and your self-esteem – so go gently!

What actually works?

In this chapter I want to show you how to set realistic and attainable goals that over time will deliver the results that you want – and let you keep them for the long-term! As we have discussed, a realistic goal should be specific and lead to a desired and attainable result through well-planned steps that are easily achievable. In addition, you should be the person setting the goal by deciding on what is most appropriate for you. You can then make your own reward system work for you during the tough times ahead – either by allowing yourself external rewards such as buying new clothes or enhancing internal rewards like the priceless feeling of accomplishment every time you achieve a goal! Note that this is a self-reinforcing process that only works with realistic goals. Too easy and you do not feel rewarded, too hard and you will become discouraged before the end. Last but not least, include regular positive feedback for yourself (e.g. by keeping a food diary and reading it) along the way, and choose to use tools that can help you such as monitoring your physical activity levels and finding social support. However, you should be aware that if you focus exclusively on the external rewards you can be very disappointed when what you expect to happen does not. For example, if you want to lose weight so that you can be admired by your peers for your hard work, it can happen that you may not get all the compliments that you crave – people are simply too busy with their own lives to notice hard-won changes in yours! However, when your motivation is rooted in both the inside and outside worlds you maximize your chances of achieving your goals because no matter what happens you can still count on yourself [43, 53].

Do what Successful Losers do!

By setting realistic and attainable goals, Successful Losers organize their intentions to change. They get more information and use it to break down their desires into several way point goals – and develop skills to enable them to attain these into practical and manageable steps.

Through setting clear goals, Successful Losers also make adjustments in other habits that facilitate their change. If their long-term goal is to lose 50 pounds by being more physically active and eating healthily, they decide to break down their goal in smaller short-term goals, targeting losing 10 pounds every two months until they reach their goal. So, in ten months they are supposed to have lost the total of 50 pounds. In order to achieve their goals, Successful Losers also carefully plan their time and actions. Instead of going directly home after work, they get off to engage in 45 min of moderate intensity cardiovascular exercise at the gym on the way home three days a week. In addition, they plan their meals ahead of time to make sure they always have healthy food at hand and decide to increase intake of fruit and vegetables to 5 portions a day.

And more, Successful Losers weigh themselves every week to make sure they are heading in the right direction. At the end of two months they have lost the planned 10 pounds. They feel proud and motivated to continue setting higher and higher goals because they know they can achieve them [43].

Now you know who the Successful Losers are and what they can teach you. You have discovered some of the reasons for why you eat as you do. And you have learned that no matter what, you are not pre-destined to be fat. Perhaps you have even decided to become a Successful Loser yourself, starting with realistic and attainable goals. It is now time to continue to Part II, where we discover the secrets that every Successful Loser knows!

Chapter 5 in a nutshell

❖ Successful Losers know that to achieve long-term goals, you need to break these down into multiple smaller, short-term ones. Most of us simply can't really be bothered about things that may or may not happen in the long-term, but we do get motivated by something in our near future.

❖ Self-knowledge is essential! Discover what motivates you to achieve your goals, and use this knowledge to keep moving towards lasting change.

❖ Do not compare yourself to others! What works for other people may not work for you!

❖ Make sure that you are the one setting your goals! Science shows that goals that you have decided on yourself are much easier to attain than those coming from outside.

❖ Successful Losers know that a good goal is specific and leads to a desired and attainable result through a number of well-planned steps that are possible.

Part II

Secrets of Successful Losers

[Secret I]

Successful Losers know they CAN lose weight

"What we can or cannot do, what we consider possible or impossible, is rarely a function of our true capability. It is more likely a function of our beliefs about who we are."

Anthony Robbins

Getting to your ideal weight and keeping the body of your dreams starts from within. By that I do not only mean literally – the food you put in your mouth – but more importantly with a genuine belief in that you can achieve your goals. Millions of people around the world want to lose weight. However, only a few actually really believe they can – and these few are the ones who succeed! The belief in yourself and your power to really change your circumstances is the first and most important step on the path to a new, healthy lifestyle. It is like building a house – you want a strong foundation, not to build on sand. Your belief in yourself is that foundation – and what a solid foundation it is! People who believe in their ability to adopt a healthy lifestyle and lose weight end up losing more weight and staying slim for longer than do people who do not [54, 55]. All Successful Losers have this faith in themselves. Accordingly, Successful Losers are optimistic about their possibility to change, focus on the many benefits of a healthier body and spend less time dwelling on past failures or making excuses than do the average dieter. While these people recognize the challenges of modern living, they are confident that they – and not some external force – control their lives and can "do it their way". Just like you and me, they face many demands on their time – jobs, children, a social life or even one or more chronic health conditions. The difference is that they knew it was possible and they knew they could make it – and they did!

"The belief in yourself and your power to really change your circumstances is the first and most important step on the path to a new, healthy lifestyle"

From a very early age, we are conditioned to accept other peoples' beliefs about ourselves. Indeed, our self-image is molded by the thousands of subtle signals we have received about what is good or bad, right or wrong from our families, teachers and friends. Some of these beliefs can be constructive and empower us – such as the belief that you always know what to do. Others can severely handicap you and become a burden if not addressed head on – by yourself or with help. Take home message? Do not believe everything that you think that you know about yourself – and definitely do not believe everything people say about you or, worse, you think they think about you! Even if your grandmother never meant to offend or harm you when she asked: "Why do you want to lose weight? You have always been the chubby one in the family – why change now?" she may have contributed to your self-image as a fat person. As hard as it is to remember such negative remarks – think back and try to figure out why you have the self-image that you do, and remember that only you can decide what to believe about yourself.

The power of our thoughts is amazing! We truly change to conform to our beliefs. For instance, in a study of fifty-four obese women, participants were divided into two groups: one group was composed of confident participants called "believers", and the other less confident group was called "disbelievers". In this study, "believers" not only had better self-esteem, but they were also more confident in their ability to reach their goals and control their weight – they felt that they "had what it takes" for weight control and were not prone to give up easily. As you can guess, being a "disbeliever" meant a lower faith in one's ability to control one's weight and a greater tendency to give up. During the following 9 months, the "believers" maintained a lower body weight than the "disbelievers". But perhaps most relevant and interesting, moving from being a "disbeliever" to becoming a "believer" during the study also improved weight loss [54].

As simple as it sounds, truly believing that you can change your life is one of the most difficult but important aids for achieving your goals. If you really believe that you can do what you want – to the point where you can actually see yourself when you close your eyes – you are one big step closer to getting there. Professional athletes have been using this technique for years! This is because they know that those sportsmen and – women who use visualization techniques to enhance their training are much more likely to win. In fact, those athletes who are the most confident in their ability to use visualization techniques are also the ones who achieve the best results [56].

I often meet clients who say that they want to lose weight, but who are unsure of their ability to do so. If that is where you are now, then you are probably not ready to lose weight yet. Indeed, as we saw in Chapter 4, change only happens when you both want it and are prepared to go for it! In the end, however hard it might be to believe now, you can decide to believe that you are a fat failure who will never lose weight. Or you can decide to believe that through your previous setbacks you now know yourself better and are therefore more prepared to make the necessary changes to achieve your goals. It really is your choice!

Successful Loser: Sabrina J.

Age: 42 years old

Weight lost: 85 pounds

Weight maintained for: 6 years

Sabrina J., a 42 years old writer, told me that despite having achieved considerable professional success, she had always had to struggle with her self-image. "I knew I was good at school and admired because of my high grades – that is how I identify myself, as a good student. I have also been taught that taking care of my physical appearance was shallow and irrelevant to being a good person – which was the perfect excuse for not practicing any sport or exercising all through high school. I must confess that back then, I considered myself intellectually above sports. I now know the truth – my looks were the least of my problems! In my mid-thirties I was hypertensive and di

abetic as a result of obesity! My doctor's blunt advice helped me to realize that I had done my body a great disservice, and that I had to do something to change!"

"I started by writing down – I'm a writer after all – the things I needed to change in my life. That included quitting smoking, cutting down on junk food and starting to move my fat ass more! I almost gave up when I saw how much I had to do, but I KNEW that I could do it. Using my list and working step-by-step, I looked up advice on weight loss websites, enrolled in a gym for women, and cut back on junk food by buying a soup maker and then baking machine –I put both in the middle of my kitchen table and forced myself to use. I think that weight loss is more of a mental battle than a physical one, once you convince yourself change is possible, you are more than halfway there. I am not saying it's easy, I spent a lot of sweat and tears, but I can now say that I am a Successful Loser. And if I can become a Successful Loser I am sure anyone can. I have achieved my goal which was to lose a massive 85 pounds and now I have adopted a healthy lifestyle to make sure that I will never gain it back!"

Tips from Successful losers:

❖ Change your inner dialogue. Do you know that voice inside of you that always makes you doubt yourself? The voice that says: "You have failed so many times, why bother trying again?" That voice is your worst enemy, and you must shut it up and replace it with a more supportive one. Try becoming your own cheerleader; cheering yourself on a daily basis will help you change your self-image. You will see incredible changes once you have crossed that mental valley and emerged with new self-confidence.

❖ Focus on and celebrate your past successes. Think of a time when you achieved a goal that you had thought difficult. How did you feel then? Reflecting on past success can increase your self-confidence and lead to a more proactive attitude in the present.

❖ Write down a list of things that you are good at. Have you always been good at those things? Or did it take you time and practice to become skilled in any of them? Weight loss is not so much about genes or luck as it is about planning, hard work and practice!

[Secret II]

Successful Losers never diet

Anonymous

To be on a diet has become the norm for a lot of people, with about six out of ten Americans claiming to be on a diet or trying to lose weight at any given time [57]. Most of these individuals (perhaps also you?) have tried dieting at some point, lost weight, but then gained it all back a little later. With so many people interested in losing weight, why is it that despite all the nutritional knowledge discovered and rediscovered over the last decades, people are still getting fatter?

For many years the word "diet" has been a mainstay of popular culture. It keeps popping up all over the place; on the cover of magazines, in the titles of books, on daytime TV shows, and as a perpetual topic of discussion in the workplaces and classrooms around the country. Even children nowadays claim to be dieting (which it is not recommended!). Despite all this hype, or perhaps because of it, little consideration has been given to what it really means "to be on a diet". A diet literally means the food and drink we consume regularly. Nowadays, we say diet only when we mean avoiding food that we usually eat. Instead of nourishment, a diet today is associated with short-term starvation in order to achieve a slimmer body. No wonder that it carries such a sacrificing connotation or that it soon becomes a huge burden to be on! So, why do so many people insist on being on a diet?

Dieting can make you fat

One of the key factors in the long-term success of a weight loss program is its ability to keep you feeling full, but at the same time reducing your calorie intake. Reducing the number of calories that you eat every day does not necessarily mean eating less food – but you do have to eat the right kinds of food. In fact, being hungry during weight loss probably means that you will regain your initial weight after a restrictive diet! Again looking to health research, when 94 college students who were both slim and fat were tested, impulsivity and hunger control influenced the body weight and food intake of every single one! But only impulsive participants bought more snacks – and only when feeling hungry [58]. So, being hungry actually inhibits you and diminishes your resolve – as you may have noticed! Considering that most diets out there promote – even celebrate – hunger instead of preventing it, it is no wonder that it so difficult to stick to a restrictive diet for long. Hence the three, ten, fourteen, etc. days diet – there has to be an end to the pain visible for anyone to risk taking on the challenge!

In the heartland of dieting, California, researchers compared two different diets – one considered restrictive and the other based on encouraging healthy eating. After one year of regular visits and diet advice, both diet groups had lost weight and improved their health. But after two years, those placed on the restrictive diet had regained all of the weight lost, while their self-esteem was lower and their health worse than before the study started! Meanwhile, most participants put on the healthy diet were still slim after two years, reported a higher self-esteem than before and had further improved their blood pressures. So, like the scientists behind the study, we must conclude that restrictive diets only serve as quick fixes whose results are hard, if not impossible, to maintain over time [59]! In my and other's experience, restrictive dieting also increases the risk of developing problematic eating patterns, such as binge eating [60, 61].

Successful Losers do not diet, but watch what they eat and aim to satisfy their hunger with the right kinds of food. It is not by chance that Successful Losers in general eat all their daily meals – but with fewer calories, smaller portions and less fat than your average dieter! Unlike most of us – failing on diet after diet – Successful Losers know better than to diet. They know there is no such a thing as being "on" or "off" a diet.

> *"Successful Losers do not diet, but watch what they eat*
> *and aim to satisfy their hunger with the right kinds of food"*

Eating healthy for Successful Losers is a lifelong commitment, not something you do for a couple of months until you lose weight and then can go back to your old ways again. However, just as for you or me, eating is a pleasurable activity for them – only they have made sure to teach themselves to find pleasure in eating a fruit salad instead of chocolate cake. Eating healthy for them is an automatic habit, like brushing their teeth or combing their hair! Importantly, a healthy diet does not mean eating salads (salads can be fat too, if you add a lot of dressing!) all the time while never touching candies. A good rule of thumb for healthy eating is 85/15. You aim to eat healthy foods 85% of the time, but 15% of the time you can eat whatever you want – in small portions, taking time to savor each bite! Contrary to most of us, Successful Losers do not see their eating habits as an all or nothing approach – they know that in order to have a healthy life and a killer body, they do not have to be perfect all the time.

Successful Loser: Michael W.

Age: 36 years old

Weight lost: 62 pounds

Weight maintained for: 5 years

Michael W., a 36 years old engineer, confessed to me that he had incessantly dieted for most of his life. In fact, he told me, "my life used to go in cycles, each one starting when one diet finished and the next started. The more I dieted the more difficult it would become to lose weight. Then, I heard of this local weight-loss program. I thought it might be a good place to meet someone. I also liked that it emphasized changing regular habits: eating more fruit and vegetables instead of processed foods, developing a physical activity routine, etc. Heck, I had tried just about everything, so decided to give this one a go too! I don't know why, guess I was just ready for change, but I went with a more rounded attitude, like this is going to be a new way of life, and this is the way I am going to live, I am not just doing this for now, it's for the rest of my life. And boy, did it work! The best thing is that unlike dieting, the longer you do it the easier it becomes!"

After losing more than 60 pounds in one year and keeping it for another 4 years, Michael W. says "That's it! I have found the magic formula to successful weight loss – focus on getting a healthy body, learn what to eat and move more. It is as simple as that!"

Tips from Successful losers:

❖ Successful Losers never diet. Dieting as it is practiced today is not healthy or sustainable – and besides, it will make you miserable!

❖ Torturing yourself with diets that promote hunger is the surest way to sabotage your attempts to lose weight. Make sure that you adopt a healthy diet that promotes satiety instead.

❖ In your new healthy eating habits, make room for your favorite foods – but make sure that you eat them in moderation!

❖ Eating healthily is a habit – the more you practice, the easier it gets. Just ask any Successful Loser!

[Secret III]

Make healthy eating a daily habit

"You are not what you eat, but what you routinely eat."

T.G. Axelsson

Have you ever thought how wonderful it would be if you could eat a good meal several times a day and still lose weight? What if I tell you that this is not only possible, but also what is advised by experts? We in the dietitian's community recommend eating three proper meals a day (breakfast, lunch and dinner), along with 2-3 small, healthy, snacks in between (a morning snack, an afternoon snack, and if you sleep late, a night snack).

Too many people insist on starving themselves to lose weight – which as we have seen does not work! The problem is that your body is smart and it notices when it has not been fed for some time (more than 4 hours). When it notices, alarm bells ring and the body enters starvation mode – which is focused on saving energy (it takes days to weeks before the body starts burning fat). Instead of losing weight, you accumulate fat to act as a reserve for when you decide to starve again! Better to make more, just in case! The take home message is this: do not starve your body to lose weight; it is a very finely tuned and fantastic machine that works better when well fed! Skipping meals only makes you fatter and hungrier – and when you are hungry it is very hard to control what you eat, resulting in you sooner or later giving up on your intention to eat healthily and gaining your weight back. This gain of weight after a diet is called the "rebound effect".

Another interesting effect that is important when trying to lose weight is the "habituation effect". This means that we get used to most things, including meals that would cause our ancestors to shake their heads in bemusement. This is well illustrated by a study with healthy adults from the US Department of Agriculture. Each participant was asked to either eat an entire day's caloric intake in one sitting, or to eat the same amount of calories divided into three daily meals. After 8 weeks of doing this (poor souls!), the group eating one huge meal not only felt hungrier than those eating three meals, but they also felt less full after their gigantic meal than did those who ate three small ones! Simply put, the one-large-meal-a-day group had gotten used to their big meal and to the time that it was served, causing them to become hungry again long before their next meal and to develop an appetite to match their large meal [62].

It turns out your mother was right when she told you to eat your breakfast so that you would grow up strong! Beyond a shadow of a doubt, breakfast really is the most important meal of the day. Successful Losers know that! That is why they never skip a meal, and especially not breakfast [63]! Breakfast breaks the starvation mode that your body enters as you sleep, helping you to reduce hunger throughout the day. Indeed, having a healthy breakfast helps you to choose low calorie foods during the rest of the day, as well as giving you energy to be physically active, two behaviors that are key to losing more weight [64].

If you are planning to lose weight and stay slim, I strongly suggest that you not only eat your breakfast every day, but also that you regularly eat your meals and snacks! Healthy snacks help you to pack extra nutrients into your day without containing too many calories. They also prevent you from becoming too hungry before the next meal, reducing your likelihood of eating too much. However, not all snacks are created equal. When snacking, choose healthy foods such as non-fat yogurt with fresh fruit, whole-grain bread with low-fat cheese, or nuts and seeds. Most importantly, avoid snacks high in calories, sugar and saturated fat. Yes, this means most sweetbreads, candies, sodas and fast-food! Even artificially sweetened products are less than ideal, as they help your tongue to stay used to large amounts of sweet taste – which means that it will react poorly to smaller amounts such as that present in an apple or other healthy snack.

Size matters – bigger is not always better!

We have been taught to believe that bigger is better; a big house is better than a small one, a big car is more comfortable than a small car, and a big bank account surplus is definitely better than a small one. However, when it comes to food, a bigger portion size is seldom the best choice. I realize that you may be used to equating size with quality and value for money, and there would be nothing wrong with a large portion size if it were not for the fact that the bigger the portion, the more you will eat. During the last decades, the portion sizes of virtually all food products (from ready-to-eat products to junk food to restaurant meals) have dramatically increased – ironically, so have our waistlines [35]. Nowadays, super-sized portions are perceived as the norm and happily consumed at one sitting – what I call portion distortion [65].

*Successful Losers know that over-sized portions trick
them into eating more than they should.*

Naturally this has consequences. For example, the larger the portion size served to children, the more they tend to overeat [66]. And not only children are affected by portion distortion! In one recent study of adults, researchers offered participants sandwiches of different sizes (but the same taste) on different days, and found that the bigger the sandwich served, the more of it was eaten [65]. Talk about eating with your eyes!
Successful Losers know that over-sized portions trick them into eating more than they should. As a countermeasure, they manage their personal environment so as to make it easier for them to eat healthily. For example, eating at home they eat on smaller plates and drink in thin tall glasses even when alone, to give their brains the impression that they are having a big portion when in reality they are not! Another commonly used trick among Successful Losers is to mentally divide their plate into two halves, with one

side of the plate always filled with only greens like salads and vegetables (no fat in this side!), the other side is mainly taken up by complex carbs and lean proteins (to learn more about complex carbs and lean proteins, see Chapter 7), with a small side of healthy fats.

But what about lunch at work or dinner with friends? For many of us, eating our meals away from home has become more the norm than an exception. The average American family today uses forty cents out of every dollar they spend on food to buy meals outside of their homes [67]. In addition, Americans are more and more moving their socializing from their homes to the restaurant [68]. Controlling portion size when eating out can be a real challenge, but that should not undermine your efforts to eat healthily. Trying to change one's eating habits does not mean that eating out is out of the question. While it is more difficult to control portion sizes when eating out, you are never forced to finish what you are served. If it is a social event, it may also be acceptable to share a dish with your friend. Or go to one of the many restaurants (including many Chinese, Japanese or Lebanese) that offer a number of plates to be shared by the whole table. Nowadays, it is easier to find places where healthy food is part of the menu. Even fast-food restaurants are offering healthy choices, including fruit or vegetables as a side-dish instead of the infamous fries, and low-fat milk or bottled water instead of soda. Even if you have got to have your fix of fast-food every now and then, do not go for the super-size options. They may seem like good value for money, but just think about how much time you are going to have to spend to burn those extra calories – not to mention the negative effects on your health.

To be a Successful Loser, you do not have to weigh and measure everything you put in your mouth (although it can definitely help!), nor do you have to give up your favorite foods. What you need to do is to learn the contents of what you eat (more on that later on the book!).

By following these tricks from Successful Losers, you also can enjoy your favorite foods – and still achieve your goals!

Successful Loser: Anne T.

Age: 40 years old

Weight lost: 55 pounds

Weight maintained for: 4 years

Anne T., a 40-year-old secretary who has lost 55 pounds over the course of two years and kept it off for the last four, told me that being dumped by her boyfriend motivated her to start losing weight. "He said that he wasn't attracted to me anymore because I was too fat. Anyway, with him gone I was all alone and needed some change! At first, I think I was mostly motivated by anger and indignation. How can someone be so insensitive and superficial? I wanted to lose the weight to make him regret that he dumped me! Then, as time passed I got over the break-up. But both my girlfriends and I noticed how good I was feeling, and how happy I was taking care of myself. For the first time in my life, I realize that I am an important person, a VIP, I am worth being taking care of!"

"As anyone who has tried to diet knows, changing a lifetime of bad habits does not happen overnight. I was no exception! I first tried various miracle cures – but they didn't work and made me feel even more of a failure. Then a friend who's a nurse recommended me to see a dietitian. I was committed to become a better version of myself, and I focused less on my weight and more on how I felt. So, I consulted the dietitian to help me understand what I needed to eat in order to lose weight. The main challenge for me was to stop ordering take-outs (read junk food) and start cooking my meals at home. I used to dislike cooking and

avoided it as much as I could. Then I started to try new recipes and experiment with new kinds of food – healthy foods that I

hadn't tried before – and I realized that I was actually a pretty good chef! Cooking can be simple, fast and tasty. I also started swimming once a week in the evenings, and walking to the carpool parking instead of driving". Now Anne T. eats breakfast every day and cooks dinner most nights of the week – and often brings the leftovers to work as lunch the next day. "Nowadays, I rarely eat junk food but when I do I make sure to order healthy side dishes and drinks – like salads with low-fat dressing or a bag of baby carrots with a bottle of sparkling water with lime. I still get to eat what I want but manage to cut a lot of the calories out of the meal." "Who knew that being dumped for being too fat would turn out to be the best thing that ever happened to me!"

Tips from Successful losers:

- ❖ Plan your eating! Eat three meals (breakfast, lunch and dinner) and two or three healthy snacks every day. Do not skip any meal – it will only make you hungrier and more vulnerable to overeating.

❖ Breakfast is the most important meal of the day. Successful Losers eat a healthy breakfast every day!

❖ Start your meals with a small serving of salad or fruit. By the time you get to the main course, you will be less hungry.

❖ Successful Losers control their portion size by using smaller plates, glasses and bowls! They also stop eating when they know that they have had enough – rather than emptying their plate. What about you?

❖ When eating out, order one appetizer for the whole table before dinner, then one dessert with multiple forks after dinner. It is a smart way to eat less *and* save money [69].

❖ When eating out, ask for a takeout box with half of your meal put in it before the meal is served. That helps you to avoid eating too much – and gets you two meals for the price of one [69].

[Secret IV]

Make physical activity a part of their lives

"Habit is stronger than nature."

Quintus Curtius Rufus

There is a lot of wisdom in the saying "use it or lose it"! Our bodies were designed for a time when survival depended on the ability to run and walk long distances to find food and shelter. Obviously, that is no longer the case, and our modern lifestyles are far from those of our ancestors. Simply put, while evolution works over thousands of years, the industrial revolution, office work and modern transport were all invented in the last 150 years or so. Consequently, most modern societies are built so as to minimize daily physical activity and help us along in our busy schedules. No wonder that an increasing number of people of all ages, sexes and ethnicities are developing some sort of chronic overnutrition (getting fatter), which in turn drives the rapid increase in lifestyle conditions such as diabetes, high blood pressure and heart disease. Many reasons are used as an excuse by people who are not physically active. Among the most popular explanations are lack of time, family obligations and lack of motivation [70]. This despite the fact that regular physical activity can prevent or improve most of the major health issues of our time.

If you stop someone on the street and ask this person what the benefits of physical activity are, I bet that she or he can answer you correctly! Indeed, even though most people know about the beneficial effects of exercise, starting and maintaining regular physical activity appear to be supremely difficult. Even those motivated to start an exercise program usually give up when confronted with unexpected events, family obligations or chaotic schedules. Almost half of American adults do not even come close to the recommended 30 minutes of physical activity on five or more days a week [71]. Worldwide, 31% of the population do not attain this activity level, while in developed countries 48% of women and 41% of men are not sufficiently physically active on a regular basis [72]. On the other hand, 72% of Successful Losers meet or exceed the minimum recommendation of physical activity [73]. You can tell where I am going with this, right?

To be physically active you do not have to enroll in an expensive gym, buy the latest fitness equipment or hire a personal trainer (although all of these options can be very helpful!). Successful Losers know that small changes in their daily routine will pay off handsomely. For example, taking the stairs instead of the elevator, walking to work, the bus or school, or finding other ways to incorporate physical movement into your daily routine can all lead to big results. Just to have an idea, during one hour of cleaning your home you burn around 250 kcal – the equivalent of walking rapidly for the same one hour!

Successful Losers are not immune to the sedentary modern life. Like most of us they often have a sedentary job and own a car or two. They face challenges similar to the ones that you face, they live in the same society as you do, also feel tired after work, and their days contain the same amount of hours as yours. Despite all that, Successful Losers "make" time to be physically active by ensuring that it is a priority. They know it is central for achieving their goals, and are better than most at creating situations to incorporate physical activity into their daily routine. For example, they will go to the gym even when they come home tired after work because that's what they always do, go for a walk even when the temperature is below freezing as they have a dog or a walking buddy that they cannot let down, or check online for a hotel with a gym or bring their running shoes when travelling! Studies have proven what Successful Losers already know, that spending more leisure time outdoors – including on activities such as cycling, walking the dog, playing with the kids or playing sports – leads to less time watching TV, surfing the internet and other sedentary activities, and consequently to more exercise [4, 74]. Overall, Successful Losers are also more likely to use the many chances to be physically active in daily life. For example, they always take the stairs instead of the elevator or escalators, often walk to another bus stop instead of to the closest one, and frequently choose a lunch spot farther from the office (and with healthier food!), affording them a midday walk.

Physical activity or exercise: what's the difference?

You may never have wondered about the difference between physical activity and exercise. More often than not, people think that physical activity and exercise are synonymous – but they are not! Here is why: physical activity is any sustained movement of the body produced through use of your muscles, and it results in energy expenditure (from a short walk to intense exercise). On the other hand, exercise is a planned, organized and repetitive bodily movement mainly performed for pleasure or health benefits [75].

"Physical activity is decisively important for losing weight and staying slim"

So, when you go to the gym and work out that's called exercise, but when you take the stairs instead of the elevator you are being physically active. It may seem like a completely academic splitting of hairs, but you can lose a lot of weight (and stay slim) even if you do not exercise. And most people who are not into intense exercise find physical activity to be less boring and more meaningful – after all, most of us need to get somewhere every day. I do not mean that exercise is not important for your general health, it is and tremendously so! Exercise is an excellent way to lose weight and to keep it off, but it is often not the first thing that someone who has committed to losing weight can appreciate – remember the setting of realistic goals discussed previously. My point is that even if you do not have the motivation, stamina or time to exercise right now, you can and should still be physically active if you want to lose weight. And once you are on track with the weight loss – regular exercise may be just the thing for you! Physical activity is decisively important for losing weight and staying slim over time [76, 77].

Amazingly, physical activity not only helps you to burn calories, but it also improves your eating habits by increasing mindful eating and decreasing hunger sensations. As if that wasn't enough, it is a great booster for your self-esteem and can improve mental health leading to that missing motivation to both continue on the road to health, and perhaps also the curiosity and self-esteem to try exercise as well [78].

Successful Loser: Phil M.

Age: 51 years old

Weight lost: 70 pounds

Weight maintained for: 8 years

Phil M., now 51 years old, works as a car salesman. He has lost an incredible 70 pounds by replacing unhealthy lifestyle habits with healthier ones. "I had gotten to the point that my weight was negatively affecting every aspect of my life. At work, I could hardly fit into a car to show it to my clients. At home, I did not have energy to do anything and my kids were always complaining that our life was boring. And my health was rapidly declining as the doctor kindly pointed out so many times."

Phil M. told me that he never really gave food much thought. He would just eat whatever was most convenient. "For example, dinner to me consisted of stopping by the nearest drive-thru and picking up some cheap, tasty and convenient food. I didn't even bother to get out of my car, let alone walk inside the restaurant! Even though I have always known of the theoretical benefits of regular physical activity, I always found some excuse to never really give it a chance. Not all fat people are lazy, but I was! Sitting on my fat ass all day avoiding any situation that required breaking a sweat."

"I say that everyone has a turning point in their lives, when they have hit bottom and really understand the simply choice – change or die! Mine came as a heart attack. As I look back and remember, what really gave me the jolt I needed to change was the panic I saw in my three boys' eyes. Since then, I have promised them and myself that I will see them grow up without them having to worry if I will be around or not."

Tips from Successful losers:

❖ Successful Losers choose to do the types of physical activity that are appropriate for their current fitness level and health goals. They identify and perform activities that they enjoy and that fit into their daily schedule.

❖   Successful Losers also work to increase their physical activity level gradually over time, to meet their personal targets and health goals.

❖   If walking is your physical activity of choice, the use of a pedometer (a small electronic device used to count steps) to track your progress can help you to maintain your activity level and motivation. Scientists advise walking at least 10 000 steps a day, but remember that you set your own goals – and sticking with them until you attain what you want is more important.

❖   Incorporate natural physical activity into your daily routine and into the activities that you perform during leisure time. That's what Successful Losers do!

❖   If you do not have time to exercise for a daily 30 minutes in one go, one solution is to divide your exercise routine into three sets of 10 minutes each throughout the day – e.g. walking 10 minutes each way to and from the bus stop, as well as walking to a lunch restaurant 5 minutes from your place of work.

❖   As always, if you have any chronic conditions and symptoms you should consult your health-care provider about the types and amounts of activity appropriate for you. Remember that very few diseases prevent you from doing any type of physical activity, while most diseases improve when you are physically active – ask your doctor about an activity that is suitable for you!

[Secret V]

Knowledge is power

"Know yourself, know your enemy!"

Sun Tzu

How will you know if you have achieved your goals? By measuring! Do not trust your feelings, or expect to wake up one day and see a new slim you in the mirror. All Successful Losers have the habit of self-monitoring. This means that they carefully and objectively observe themselves and their behavior as a way to increase awareness and motivation. Self-monitoring means that you know what you do, how you do it, and the circumstances around these behaviors [4, 79]. Self-monitoring does not mean obsessing about every calorie, weighing yourself every hour of the day or constantly comparing your looks or physical ability to those of others! Instead of draining their energies and self-esteem through useless comparisons, Successful Losers know that losing weight is a science and self-monitoring one of the best tools to steer you right. Measuring your body weight, waist circumference, food intake, exercise routine and results all give you valuable clues to unlocking your body's secrets for losing weight and staying slim [6, 80, 81].

Remember, though, that most useful information appears when you look at patterns, rather than individual measurements. So make sure to record all of your gathered data in the same place (I prefer a computer spreadsheet, because it allows me to make graphs). All Successful Losers use regular, planned self-measurements to judge the relative success of ongoing weight-loss behaviors. Knowing the facts help them to observe if months of a new behavior is working for them and for their bodies – both practically and results-wise [4].

You would do well to follow their example, as to successfully change behavior you need to constantly pay attention to your own actions, as well as to the conditions under which they occur and their direct and long-term effects [82]. Do you tend to eat more healthily at work or at home? Do you follow your exercise routine more in summer or winter? As always when dealing with yourself, successful self-monitoring depends in part on being truthful, in part on being thorough and consistent, and in part on how often you self-monitor the right measurement in relation to a desired target behavior [79, 82]. It is obviously not easy to judge the success of a new running routine if you only measure your arm circumference in the hope of detecting bigger biceps! So what to measure, and how? Read on and find out.

Self-monitoring food consumption

Self-monitoring your food consumption is commonly performed in the nutrition field by making a food diary. Food diaries are the dietitian's best friend! They are tremendously useful tools to understand what you are actually eating, when and why. But they only work if you are honest with yourself and consistent with your note-taking. A typical food diary usually entails recording what foods and drinks you actually consumed immediately after every meal, including the approximate amount, the situation and setting of the meal, your mood as well as whatever else you think may be important for your eating behavior – for example, with whom the meal was consumed. Self-monitoring food intake like this is greatly associated with success in losing weight [83-86]. Also, those whose self-monitoring records are the most complete lose more weight than those who are less thorough. And consistency in self-monitoring food intake also leads to greater weight loss [83-85]. In addition, those who lose weight only to regain it later usually decrease their self-monitoring with time – while the opposite is true for those who maintain their weight loss. Basically, the non-Successful Losers are unable to maintain the state of consciousness and dedication needed to maintain their positive behavioral changes over time, noting and correcting any slippage. Perhaps they had not prepared enough for the road ahead (including not read this book)! As a consequence, their weight climbed back up as their old habits returned. The Successful Losers, however, are much more conscious about their dietary and physical activity patterns, and consequently make more informed decisions regarding food selection, weight control and physical activity [63, 87].

Self-monitoring physical activity

Self-monitoring your physical activity over time is also a great motivator to keep going. Studying such monitoring, scientists asked participants to record their daily exercise type and duration for 6 months. Those who monitored their exercise levels not only achieved greater weight loss, but also reported having an easier time doing exercise, and exercised more often [88]. Today there are numerous free or inexpensive electronic tools that make measuring exercise easier than ever before – whether you keep the results to yourself or post them online.

Successful Losers are better than most at self-monitoring their physical activity levels. They often use a pedometer or cell phone application as a way of monitoring how much they walk or run. Those who regularly use a pedometer considerably increase their physical activity compared to previous levels. Having a step goal (such as 10 000 steps – the current recommendation) is linked to a decrease in weight [89-91 92].

If you are the gym type, a good way to keep track of your exercise routine is taking notes on how much weight you can lift, the estimated calories burned reported by various gym equipment, the numbers of sets and repetitions performed, etc. Successful Losers know that the more they know, the easier it will be for them to lose weight – and the more calories they burn during exercise, the more calories they can safely eat.

Self-monitoring your weight

Weighing yourself every hour of the day, or indeed now and then when you feel bad, is not a clever strategy – and it is definitely not self-monitoring as practiced by Successful Losers. But weighing yourself on a regular basis can help to increase awareness of your weight and its relation to food intake and physical activity. For example, regular daily weighing is linked to weight loss, while the opposite is true for less frequent weighing. Additionally, when monthly, weekly, and daily self-weighing are compared, all result in weight loss, but more frequent self-weighing is associated with a greater weight loss. In addition, weighing oneself at least once a week is needed to benefit, anything less than that only has an insignificant effect [93] [94]. Not surprisingly, a massive 75% of Successful Losers weigh themselves at least once per week [7].

"Successful self-monitoring depends in part on being truthful, in part on being thorough and consistent, and in part on how often you self-monitor"

I advise you to keep track of your weight by weighing yourself on a scale just once a week. Despite the studies suggesting that daily body weighing may lead to greater weight loss, I believe that body weight will always vary slightly from one day to the next, especially in women due to their menstrual cycle, and also depending on the time of day (before or after a meal), water intake and recent physical activity.

Tools for self-monitoring

Thanks to technological advancement, there are now many fun ways to measure your progress. Besides the great many apps and sites already available, I foresee even more tools designed specifically for self-monitoring. You can already use your smartphone to monitor not only your food intake, physical activity level and weight, but also your sleep time and quality, heart rate, pulse, etc. Several websites also allow you to monitor these things, and then help you to post everything from food intake to calorie expenditure online for all to see. Usually, these tools are free, and provide an easy way to save and study your data. If you are always on the go and own a smartphone, you can literally have your self-monitoring device with you wherever you go. For those who are more old-fashioned, or simply do not have use for a computer in their pocket, a notebook with carefully recorded data is still just as good a way of self-monitoring – sometimes better as it requires more dedication, which spills over onto your efforts at changing your habits. Regardless of the method used, the results are virtually the same as long as you are honest, consistent and detailed in your records [95].

Successful Loser: Jennifer P.

Age: 23 years old

Weight lost: 50 pounds

Weight maintained for: 2 years

Jennifer P., a 23 years old college student, told me how having an unrealistic weight target took the pleasure out of her life: "Unfortunately, I am a perfectionist. When I have a goal in mind I will do my utmost to achieve it – and feel like a failure if I do not. When it comes to my weight, it was all or nothing: I either worked very hard trying and failing to achieve my own imagined ideal body weight, or I did not care what I ate at all and consequently put on a lot of weight. To make things worse, I kept making the mistake of setting a target weight that was too low for me. Trying to get to and maintain this weight made me feel like I had no life at all. After a while, I always ended up defeated and feeling bad about myself – which is when I started overeating again, gaining the weight back. I just didn't seem to realize that not all of us are meant to look like supermodels". "Then, I realized that I was only wasting my time by yo-yo dieting again and again. Through counseling, I came to terms with the fact that I am a big boned woman who will never be skinny or have an hourglass waist. So, instead of starving myself, I started focusing on what message I was actually sending my body through food I was eating and how much of it. I noticed that my diet was mostly processed foods rich in empty calories and poor in nutrients. The next step was to keep a food diary and monitor my physical activity level. Soon, I figured out what I was doing wrong! I used to skip breakfast, snack on junk food, eat whatever lunch I could buy cheaply nearby – and to make matters worse I did not move at all! Nowadays, I eat a healthy breakfast every day even if it is on the go, I have cut down very much on the processed food and replaced it with healthier choices, and bought a pedometer to count how many steps I walk per day (over the last 18 months, I have gone from an average 2 371 steps/day to be well on my way to reaching the recommended 10 000 steps/day). After losing 50 pounds and

keeping her weight at 160 lbs for her 5'10" frame for more than two years, Jennifer P. says that "I still don't fit into the beauty ideal of glossy magazines, but I have learned that setting realistic goals and learning to love yourself, as I have, is far more attractive!"

Tips from Successful losers:

❖ Successful Losers self-monitor themselves, and keep doing it even after having achieved their goals. That is why they are so successful at keeping their weight off!

❖ Successful Losers not only monitor regularly and carefully, they also regularly follow up on their monitoring by carefully looking for lessons to be learned in all of their data. Some use computers to draw graphs, others graph on paper or simply tabulate numbers and calculate averages. The important thing is that you do not waste all of your hard-won information!

❖ There are a wide variety of ways to self-monitor. Find one (or two) that works for you – and stick with it!

❖ As a minimum, keep a food diary (either in digital or paper form), including notes on your moods and the setting of meals. Soon, you will be more aware of your eating habits and what triggers overeating in you.

❖   If you decide to weigh yourself, it is recommended that you always do it at the same time of the day and on the same day of the week to be able to compare measurements. For example, every Monday morning at 7 am, before breakfast.

❖   Remember: knowledge is power! The more you know about your lifestyle and habits, the more power you will have to change what you do not like.

[Secret VI]

Have patience and plan for the long-term

"One who can have patience can have what one will."

Benjamin Franklin

We live in a society of instant gratification. Every day, we are bombarded with the message that we have to get what we want when we want it, and it had better be fast! We have gotten used to things happening in the blink of an eye or the touch of a button. If you are like most people, you want things to happen immediately, or you lose interest – just think about what happens when your internet connection is a bit slow!

A Successful Loser knows that everything in life is a matter of perspective – short versus long-term perspective. Successful Losers consequently work on resisting immediate temptations to achieve long-term goals such as a slimmer body, increased attractiveness and better health [96]. While long-term benefits often seem less appealing in the here and now, Successful Losers know that denying immediate rewards presented pays off handsomely. Science tells us that being able to ignore short-term rewards in order to gain better long-term outcomes is a trait that predisposes you to a higher probability of success when attempting lifestyle changes [96].

"Everything in life is a matter of perspective – short versus long-term perspective."

As we have learnt, most dieters fail to lose weight or soon return to their previous weight, mainly through a lack of commitment. As I see it, this lack of commitment is often due to conflicting feelings about what they want right now and what they want in the long term. For example, you may claim to want to lose weight, but at the same time not be willing to give up your current unhealthy diet. Indeed, you might even consider changing your habits temporarily, but then go back to your old lifestyle as soon as you have reached your goal, thinking that you now deserve a short-term reward for your short-term effort. If this is you, go back and re-read the chapter on the psychology of change – perhaps you have not prepared the ground enough before attempting change?

Rewarded now or forever?

I and everyone else know that changing your lifestyle is not as easy as pressing a button! The journey to achieve your new healthy self or your dream body is not smooth and fast. It definitely requires restraint and denial of instant gratification to achieve your long-term goals. For example, rational food decisions require valuing the tradeoff between instant gratification versus the longer-term gain of health and wellness. This would seem like an easy choice, but this kind of rational food decision is very uncommon, with most of us going through our life habitually doing the same things over and over, while sometimes succumbing to distraction, lack of time, or peer pressure [97].

Next time before indulging in an unhealthy treat, I want you to stop for a second and ask yourself if succumbing to this momentary pleasure now is more important than reaching your goals. Let's say your goal is to lose 30 pounds in six months. To achieve this goal, you plan to eat more healthily and go to the gym four times a week. One day after work, you come home and as usual you are tired and a bit hungry. To achieve your goal you know that you should follow your plan and go to the gym anyway, even though at the moment you really feel like eating some chocolate chip cookies in front of the TV. You rationalize that you have worked hard today, and deserve to finally do something to relax and indulge yourself. At the same time, you can feel the guilt that will follow your diet of cookies. At this point, you ask yourself: Is eating a package of cookies in front of the TV more important than achieving my goals? In the short-term, you may think so, but after considering the situation, you realize that going to the gym (denying yourself some instant pleasure) will get you closer to your goal of losing 30 pounds, not make you feel guilty and perhaps get rid of some of that tiredness that you are feeling. In the medium-term (that is, tomorrow) you will actually feel happier and more proud of yourself for sticking to your plan, while still keeping on track to achieving the long-term benefits that you long. Not such a hard choice once you get your logical mind working, right?

Does this scenario sound familiar to you? If you are like most people, I bet it does! The best way to remain focused is to consistently think about your long-term goals and the pleasure they will bring. To lose weight, you must always manage to keep in mind that every action you take is a choice – even if that choice is made far from your conscious and logical brain. But you should also take into consideration that a life of unhealthy eating habits will not change overnight. Sometimes, even the most Successful Loser makes a wrong move. But they quickly get back on track, because they know that to have the body of their dreams, the fitness level of an athlete or the energy levels of a teenager. You must actively decide that indulging in a moment of pleasure is less pleasurable than fitting into your old pants, turning heads when you walk down the street, or being able to stop taking blood pressure medication.

Yes, you have to go through short-term discomfort. Your current body is the result of the choices you have made in the past – so to change your future, you need to start making better decisions now!

Reinforce long-term benefits!

Reinforcement is what you feel after taking an action – and the sooner after the behavior you get this feedback, the stronger it will affect you! While negative enforcement such as shame and guilt are powerful forces that help shape our social awareness, they are also great drains of energy and self-esteem. So stop guiltily overeating and burning with shame! Instead, the best thing you can do is to focus on creating new healthy habits and to reinforce these using positive cues. By focusing on the positives, praising yourself daily for any real progress, and keeping a look-out for the beneficial effects of weight loss (including improvements in your life quality, increased energy and zest, better physique, happier moods, increased self-confidence, and long term health [7]). You will feel more motivated and encouraged to continue these actions and progressing toward your goals. Reinforce good decisions, but avoid dwelling (or, worse, wallowing) on the bad. This focus will help you to avoid short-term distractions – if you really are ready to change!

Successful Loser: Nina R.
Age: 34 years old
Weight lost: 56 pounds
Weight loss maintained for: 3 years

Nina R., a 34 years old school teacher who lost 56 pounds over a period of 12 months, is a perfect example of someone who felt unable to control herself when confronted with certain foods. "I used to joke with my friends that I was a sweet junkie. I just loved anything sweet – whether it was chocolate, ice-cream or cake. Whenever I was stressed, hungry or bored I got my sugar fix. I remember once when I was in the middle of a PTA meeting at the school. The only thing I could think of was what I was going to eat when the meeting was over." Nina R. confesses to feeling ashamed of keeping a few packets of M&Ms in the glove compartment of her car. "It was so embarrassing when others found out that I hid sweets in my car, because I and they both knew that I should not be eating all the time".

"I must say it was not easy to change my relationship with food. What really set it off was seeing one of the parents at work drop their girl off in a specially built car for obese people. I realized that I could never live like that! Back then I really thought that food was my best friend, something that would always be there to comfort me.

I read a lot of books, and finally figured out that I was ready for change – and how to go about it! Now, while I still have to be vigilant about what I eat, I keep a food diary, and with it I have finally learned to differentiate my emotional needs from my hunger. I know that indulging in comfort food every time I am stressed, bored, happy, sad or frustrated will not help me to achieve my long-term goal of being healthy and happy!"

Tips from Successful losers:

❖ Think about the big picture. How do you want to look and feel in a few months? Are your actions now bringing you closer to your goal or further from it?

❖ Successful Losers focus on the long-term benefits of achieving their goals as being the best reward for their efforts. What about you?

❖ Make a list of the short-term costs and the long-term benefits of your current behaviors regarding food and physical activity. Are they bringing you closer to achieving your goals? See for yourself what you have to gain if you succeed in making the change for good.

Action	Short-term cost	Long-term benefit
Eat a healthy breakfast every day	Wake up 15 minutes earlier everyday	Be slim and healthy

[Secret VII]

Successful Losers do not blame others for their shortcomings

"You are the master of your destiny, the captain of your soul."

William Ernest Henley

Who is the boss? You are! Successful Losers know that they have what it takes to achieve their goals. They are responsible for their own lives and do not blame others or circumstances for their misfortunes. As we discussed in Secret I, Successful Losers have acquired a strong inner belief in their capacity to achieve whatever they set their minds to. In addition, Successful Losers often have an easier time than most of us making commitments and making up their minds. Studies confirm that taking responsibility for your life is important for weight management, and have shown that

Successful Losers subsequently attribute their successes to their own determination, skills, and patience [98].

You really are the boss!

In medical literature, the extent to which control over one's life is experienced as internal or external is called the locus of control. Most people tend to have one of the two. Those who have an internal locus of control believe that their lives are a consequence of their own actions and therefore that it is possible for them to influence how the future will turn out. On the other hand, those who have an external locus of control tend to believe that life is determined by fate, chance, luck, or under the control of powerful others [99].

To me, this makes a lot of sense. An internal locus of control helps you to believe that change is possible, that you are in fact responsible for making it happen. People with an internal locus of control have more confidence in the value of weight loss behaviors, while those with an external locus of control tend to believe that external factors are responsible for their overweight – and that behavioral change is only slightly useful [100]. Not surprisingly, individuals with an external locus of control also perceive more barriers to performing regular physical activity and are more dissatisfied with the social support that they received during their weight loss attempts [100].

In addition, when Successful Losers, overweight individuals and weight regainers (those who had lost a lot of weight, but then regained it) are asked about why they became overweight in the first place, they usually give very different answers. As you can guess, those that are still overweight are much more likely to attribute their weight to a medical condition and/or genes, while Successful Losers tend to identify their former behaviors as the most important cause [101]. At the extreme end of denial, severely obese people studied after they had failed to lose weight even after obesity surgery (gastric banding) sometimes claimed that they were not aware that any effort on their part was needed to lose weight after the surgery [102].

"Those who have an internal locus of control believe that their lives are a consequence of their own actions"

Unfortunately, in my practice, I often hear clients blame their obesity on genetic predisposition, a preexisting health condition, an unhelpful spouse, or even on the junk food manufacturers! Yes, it is true that all of those factors can make you fat, but only if you let them! For example, blaming your parents for bad genes that make you fat may seem logical, especially if your mother or father (or both) is overweight. But science offers a startling rebuttal: only a tiny handful of obese individuals suffer from genetic mutations that lead to obesity! Unless you have been diagnosed with such a condition (which usually requires special medical attention), I strongly suggest that you do what Successful Losers do: stop making excuses and start taking responsibility for your actions! By taking control of your life, I do not mean that you should become a control freak and obsess about every single aspect of your day – or feel shame at every lapse. However, success is entirely up to you, and you need to find constructive strategies to achieve your goals. Take control of your meals by planning your eating and shopping wisely, controlling portion size and calorie content. In addition, you need to practice to control even unpredictable situations such as unhealthy food offered in your workplace, dealing with pressures from others, and habitually exercise even in bad weather!

If you are despairing at this point – think of the future rewards! The power in making these simple changes has been proven by science [103]. Amazingly, when taught the basic strategies found in this book as part of a study, clients at some of the most renowned weight loss centers in the country continued to lose weight long after the end of the study! It is simple, really – people who take charge of their eating and exercise habits lose weight and keep it off. These are very encouraging findings; if others can do it, I bet you can do it too!

Successful Loser: Carlo L.
Age: 37 years old
Weight lost: 80 pounds
Weight maintained for: 5 years

Carlo L., a 37 years old bus driver who has lost 80 pounds, told me about how he lost his overweight in 18 months, and how he has now been keeping it off for more than 5 years. "I have always been able to find reasons to justify my obesity. First, both my mother and father are overweight, so I blamed the bad genes they passed on to me. Second, I suffer from hypothyroidism, which makes my metabolism slower than normal (although not when I am taking my medication, which

I have been since I was 30). Third, all my friends were either overweight or obese, so being fat was the norm as far as I was concerned. On top of this, I work as a bus driver so my days consist of me sitting down on my ass!" Still, after hitting the 330 pound mark (distributed over his 5'7" body frame), and developing diabetes and high blood pressure, Carlo L. heard

from the doctor that he had to lose weight if he wanted to live to old age. But that was not enough to motivate him. "I told the doctor: 'Ok, you have your opinion and I have mine. If I feel fine, it must mean I am fine!'" "But then one day I was rushed to the hospital with a hypertensive crisis – a blinding headache and chest pain. This time, I did not even have the courage to look the doctors in the eye. I knew what I had to do. That was the day I committed to change my life. But what to do, when I had been stuffing my face for all these years – I had no idea of what a healthy life looked like! At first, changing my life was not easy – it was slow, painful and frustrating, but as I stopped playing the victim and started feeling responsible and in charge of my life I realized that change was possible, and I could actually succeed! Little by little, I noticed that some of the things that I did really worked, which gave me new strength. Two of my closest friends also decided to lose weight, and we have been helping each other to maintain our new lifestyles."

"So for me, it's actually been mostly about feeling better about myself day by day that has done it, and this is a feeling that only you can give to yourself – nobody else can do it for you! Once you accept that, you have got to do what it takes to achieve your goals even if it is hard, and even if nobody believes in you – not even yourself. You still have to keep going."

Tips from Successful losers:

❖ Successful Losers do not blame others for their shortcomings! They take responsibility for their own lives.

❖ Plan ahead! Losing weight is not an easy task, but it gets much easier if you have a good plan and ready strategies to deal with common problems.

❖ Focus on the solutions, not on the problems! Successful Losers look for a solution that depends only on them – that is possible to turn into a habit – and allows them to track how well the problem is solved. Don't have time to go to the gym? A workout DVD used at home along with an exercise diary and incrementally ratcheting up the difficulty level may be the solution for you.

❖ Make your environment work for you! It is much easier to eat healthily if you keep healthy food at home, just like it is more likely that you will exercise if you leave your gym bag in the car. You never know when you can take a longer lunch break, do a power-walk, or accompany a friend to play ball!

[Secret VIII]

Focus on the solution – not on the problem

"Impossible only means that you haven't found the solution yet."

Anonymous

In an ideal world, you would have plenty of time to go out shopping for fresh ingredients to cook delicious low-fat meals. The cafeteria at work would only serve cheap, delicious and healthy foods. Fast-food would not appeal to your taste buds, nor would it ever tempt your intentions to eat healthily. There would be no stress in your life, and your colleagues would be like a perfect family, always looking after your best interests. Exercise would be fun, and a spontaneous activity, something that you look forward to. Your children, spouse or family would all listen patiently to you and then do exactly what you ask them. How easy life would be if everything worked like this to help you achieve your goals! Unfortunately, as you know life is not so simple – and most of the time to get what you want, you have to find ways around a score of obstacles thrown up by your daily life and its demands.

"You do not have to revolutionize the world to achieve your goals; you only need to revolutionize your personal circumstances!"

You may be thinking, remembering Chapter 3, that the obesogenic environment we live in makes controlling our diets almost impossible. Or that your genes make it inevitable that you are overweight. Indeed, how can you as an individual possibly hope to win the battle against overweight when our entire society seems destined to be fat? The good news is that you do not have to revolutionize the world to achieve your goal of a healthy body; you only need to revolutionize your personal circumstances! By this, I mean that you should look for ways to make your daily life healthier in the environment you live in – rather than dreaming of a perfect world. That is what every Successful Losers does!

After years of hearing a lot of excuses for why it is so difficult to lead a healthy lifestyle, I have compiled some of the most common excuses and some great solutions for you to use on yourself when you feel discouraged!

"I don't know what foods to buy/cook/eat"

Savvy food shopping

Eating healthily starts in the supermarket aisles! It is almost impossible to have a healthy diet unless you (a) cook at home most days, and (b) keep healthy foods in the fridge and unhealthy ones out of your home! For example, it is much more difficult to resist fatty food if you keep them around the house. As they say, "out of sight is out of mind!"

Never shop for groceries while you are hungry! That simple trick is one of the most powerful that I can teach you. When you are hungry, you are more likely to be impulsive, and you run the risk of filling your cart/kitchen with less than healthy food that you will probably then end up eating – starting with the candy bar in the car on the way home. Again, science supports what common sense tells us! In a study of 94 university students, hunger was the most powerful determining factor for impulsive buying of food, especially unhealthy snack foods [58]. Successful Losers know that! That is why they usually make a shopping list and have a healthy snack before going grocery shopping! Not only will you be less inclined to buy impulsively and therefore to eat unhealthily, but you will also save money if you stick to your carefully prepared list instead of falling for the "buy 1 get 1 free" offer that screams at you when you enter the store

Once you make it to the supermarket armed with your shopping list and a full stomach, it is time to pack your shopping cart with healthy items! Too many people do not know how to distinguish healthy food from junk food. If that is true for you, don't be discouraged! By learning to read food labels, you will be well on your way to healthier eating. Food labels were created to help consumers like us to make educated choices, but they are not always easy to understand and put to good use. The Food and Drug Administration offers detailed information on how to better understand what food labels say [104]. A good place to start when looking at a food label is in the nutritional facts section. There, you will find the serving size and the amount of servings in the package; usually given in familiar units such as pieces, cups or ounces/grams. After you find out how much a package contains, you should evaluate the amount of calories per likely serving – that is, how much you expect to eat (which is often a lot more than the food manufacturer expects you to eat). A serving with 40 calories or less is considered low-caloric, a serving around 100 calories is moderately caloric, while a serving of 400 calories or more is considered highly caloric. Below the calorie content are displayed the nutritional contents (fats, cholesterol, sodium and carbs). Most people eat enough of all of these without checking – and often too much! Indeed, all nutrients should be eaten in moderation, since overeating is linked to an increased risk of chronic disease such as high blood pressure, cancer and heart disease. However, there are nutrients that most Americans do not get enough of, including vitamins A, B, C, and D, dietary fiber, calcium and iron.

At the bottom of the label you will often find footnotes, among the most common of which are information on how much of your recommended daily intake is contained in a serving (remember that this may be different from what you eat). Here you may see recommended dietary intakes for several nutrients, including fats, sodium and fiber. However, look carefully and you will see that the percentage daily value (%DV) is calculated for a diet of 2 000 calories/day – which may not be what you are eating. Regardless, you can still use the percentages as reference values. If the daily value is 5 % or less, it is considered low; if it is 20% or more, it is considered high. Remember, if you eat more than one serving you have to multiply the percentage value by the number of servings.

If you are trying to lose weight, it is a good idea to avoid foods that are rich in calories, fats (especially saturated and trans-fats), sodium and sugar. Instead, try to buy those that are high in dietary fiber, vitamins and minerals. These include whole-wheat cereals, non-fat milk and yogurt, fruit and vegetables. It takes a little practice, but once you get the hang of it, you will see changes in your health and body appearing as if by magic.

"I don't have time to cook"

Plan your meals – cook your own "fast-food"

Who said that all fast-food is unhealthy? It is true that most food bought in fast-food restaurants as well as most ready-to-eat supermarket meals are not healthy. But with a little bit of planning and commitment, you can cook your own delicious and nutritious fast-food at home. Indeed, I bet that once you get the hang of it, it takes you barely as much time to prepare these foods as it does to buy ready-made food outside! Yet home-cooked is cheaper, healthier and can be made in large quantities and frozen for use as a lunchbox. For example, to prepare an oven grilled salmon with vegetables that is rich in protein, fibers, and healthy fats you don't need to spend more than 25-30 minutes. Furthermore, compared to people who report eating fast-food two or more times per week, those who report not eating fast-food at all are the ones who lose weight and stay slim [105]. That is why I recommend you to cook at least two meals (breakfast and dinner) at home every day.

Life can be unpredictable, but that does not mean your diet has to be a constant surprise! With a little planning, you can make sure that you and your family are well fed and also save money. Planning meals and measuring food are on the top of the Successful Losers' list of common healthy habits [106]. If you are not at all comfortable in the kitchen, start by trying easy recipes that do not require a lot of skills. If you don't have time to cook in the mornings or for lunch, try preparing an extra serving or more at dinner the night before and take it with you the next day. If you know that you will not be able to get healthy food in your workplace or school, you should plan ahead and bring a healthy meal with you every day! Yes, that might involve a little more work than just ordering whatever the cafeteria serves, but changing your habits through a conscious effort and patience will prolong your life and make you richer. Successful Losers know that by cooking their meals, they can control the portion size as well as the nutrient composition.

"I am not the sporty type of person"

Keep on moving

You may not have been the captain of your high school football team, or the track and field star of your school. Maybe you have never thought of yourself as the sporty type of person, and because of that you have been avoiding situations that make you sweat. Sport to you may be only something people do on TV, a very distant reality not present in your life. How is this working for you? I bet it is not working so well, or you would not be reading this book!

Even if you have never practiced any sport in your life – and going to the gym is just something that you have heard of – you can still find ways to be physically active without having to belong to a team or enroll at your local gym (although these things are highly recommended!). Remember what we discussed about the differences between exercise and physical activity? Compared to the rest of us, Successful Losers are more likely to engage in physical activity for at least 30 minutes per day and to add physical activity to their daily routine [106]. Yes, most Successful Losers do practice some type of sport – if nothing else because it makes them feel good about their new, fit body. But they also know that there are many fun ways to be more physically active without even seeming to! Real-life alternatives from my interviews include dancing in your living room, walking the dog, playing with your kids outside, walking instead of driving when practical, or whatever else you can think of that makes your heart rate go up! Successful Losers face challenges similar to the ones faced by you in your daily life. The difference is that they focus on solutions, not problems. They know what they have to do, because they have done their homework, and they create solutions that will lead them to their goals – even it means sweating from time to time. That is how they become so successful!

Successful Loser: Sarah H.
Age: 43 years old
Weight lost: 50 pounds
Weight loss maintained for: 6 years

Sarah H., a 43 years old mother of two, is a good example of how a little bit of planning can go a long way. She has lost 50 pounds by rethinking the way she eats. In her words "I just ate whatever was easier, I never really thought about what was in the food". After being diagnosed as a diabetic, she started thinking about what she was doing to herself (and to her kids). After the first shock, she realized that if she wanted to live a long and healthy life she had to change her diet. "We used to have junk food for dinner most nights of the week, it was easy and the children liked it. Nowadays, we have turned dinnertime into a fun family activity where everyone does a little to help cook dinner. It took some time to get used to this new routine, but we eventually got the hang of it. Now, junk food is only for special occasions, and I can tell from my kids that they feel better for it!"

Tips from Successful losers:

❖ Successful Losers acknowledge the challenges, but focus on finding solutions! They plan their new, healthier lives, making sure that they have the right information.

❖ Never go grocery shopping hungry! You will end up impulsively buying a lot of unhealthy food that you should not be eating.

❖ Plan your trips to the supermarket! Do not go grocery shopping before making a list of the things you need to buy. It will save you time and money!

❖ Read food labels before you buy your food – not at home around the kitchen table. That way, you can make sure to buy only items that are low in calories, low in fats (especially saturated and trans fats) and sodium – but rich in proteins, vitamins, minerals and fibers. Avoid as much as possible foods with added sugar – whether it be called glucose, fructose or galactose!

❖ Eat more home-cooked meals! Not only are they healthier, but they also save you money when compared to eating out.

❖ Successful Losers know that they are surrounded by an obesogenic environment, and because of this they micromanage certain things by planning their meals, creating situations that force them to be more physically active, and most importantly, they stick to their plans even when they feel like quitting!

❖ Successful Losers find fun and creative ways to be physically active. What about you?

[Secret IX]

Successful Losers are surrounded by people who help them to keep their empowering habits

"Man is a social animal."

Baruch Spinoza

No man or woman is an island! From the moment we are born, we need others to develop and learn about the world around us. Our connections to others are fundamental not only for survival, but also in most cases for health and happiness.

When Harvard researchers decided to study how obesity is spread in our environment, they were surprised to discover that obesity can be transmitted almost as a contagious disease through our social network [24] That is, our personal relationships – with friends, family members or spouse – can contribute to our body weight! According to this study, if you have a friend who becomes obese

126

your risk of becoming obese increases by 57%. If the same happens to one of your siblings, the probability that you will become obese increases by 40%. And more, if your spouse becomes obese, the chance that you will become obese too increases by 37%. Luckily, it seems that your neighbors' waistline does not impact yours (unless you are very good friends with your neighbor!). This study also suggests that your close social circle influences your body weight more than your geographic location. As they say, you are the company you keep!

"Obesity can be transmitted almost as a contagious disease through our social network"

But are social surroundings so important when changing lifestyle to a healthier one? I would argue that it is definitely one of the most influential determinants of our behaviors – because that is what evolution has taught us. Adapt, belong and survive! And you can use this to your advantage – by using the powerful forces of social support to help you! Social support is often said to mean a relationship between two or more individuals involving emotional concern (esteem, affect, trust, concern); influential aid (aid in kind, money, labor); appraisal (affirmation, feedback); and information exchange (advice, suggestion). Social support facilitates initial weight loss and then helps to maintain a healthy body weight [4, 107, 108]. In the battle to lose weight, your social support groups – that's your spouse or partner, your friends, and even your acquaintances and colleagues at work – are uniquely important as aids [109]. Regardless of if you belong to a declared support group, a weight loss pact, a buddy system or if you just listen to feedback from your family, social support leads to better results [80, 81, 110]. Successful Losers know the great importance of their social network for getting what they want – including a sexy body! But how do you go about this? What should you do if your closest friends, family members or spouse either don't think your overweight is a problem, or are themselves obese? Should you avoid them like the plague? Of course not, that is not only prejudicial, but also inhumane and stupid! What would Successful Losers do in this situation? Read on and you will discover the answer!

Your significant other – friend or foe?

Your significant other, should you have one, is your most important ally in reaching your goals. Not only do they influence your everyday choices in thousands of little ways, but they can also support you – or not – by both their words, and more importantly, by modifying their lifestyle to support you in making the necessary changes to achieve your goals. In a study with Successful Losers, participants who had spouses or friends that joined them in their weight loss program reported that these partners acted as confidants and supporters [111]. However, the opposite can also be true. In the same study, Successful Losers reported that it was not uncommon for their social group (spouses, family and friends) to make mean comments such as, "you look ill after you have lost weight", "stop being so fussy with everything" or "I don't think you should lose any more weight" – as well as downplaying or discouraging their efforts to continue their healthy habits [111]. Despite their best intentions or otherwise, your loved ones may actually be sabotaging your efforts to achieve your goals. This lack of support can of course be due to many causes, but some important ones are likely to be feelings of jealousy, the fear that your relationship might change when your body changes, or the impact that your choices can have on a shared lifestyle [112]. Regardless, before you start changing lifestyle, and often after, I suggest that you talk to your social support group about it. Explain your reasons for wanting to change, how important their support is to you, and ensure them that you still be the same person, but slimmer and more energetic!

This is exactly what Successful Losers do! They persuade those closest to them to become their allies in the journey to a healthier and happier life. When comparing Successful Losers with weight regainers the former are much more likely to seek social support from family and friends, as well as to seek professional guidance, when dealing with life's challenges – including their weight problems. Meanwhile, weight regainers are not only more reluctant to seek help, but are also very good at ignoring or denying their problems even when well intentioned family or friends offer to help them [63].

Peer pressure matters!

Life is more enjoyable when we share it with others! In good times and bad, having the support of others can make challenges seem less intimating and encourage you to follow through on your plans. When it comes to losing and maintaining weight, having a strong support group can take you a long way.

In fact, in health science research whether study participants are recruited alone or with friends can affect their weight loss! In some studies, those recruited with friends, or who receive social support as part of their program, lose more weight and stay slimmer for longer than those going at it alone [113]. In one case, social support led to a whopping 66% maintaining their full weight loss to the end of the study! So if you can, bring a friend, spouse or colleague along with you when embarking on your weight loss journey! And if you can't, you can still benefit from social support by finding a buddy along the way! A buddy is someone – a new acquaintance, old friend, casual encounter or even a strictly online relationship – who is working to achieve goals similar to yours. A buddy system simply means a friendship where you two help each other to succeed by offering emotional, motivational and strategic support. Having a buddy can be very beneficial when attempting positive behavioral change, and is probably less taxing on your close friendships [114].

Online help – get connected

With the world becoming more and more connected – think e-mail, blogs, Twitter, Facebook, etc. – new channels for social support abound. If in the past it would take days for you to receive a letter, you can now communicate with a diet buddy in virtually any part of the world almost instantaneously. As geographic distances have shrunk, your chances of finding friends and support have greatly improved, especially if you live outside a big city. Nowadays, social support is also available in many different forms. Online social networks for weight loss support offer forums and web communities, as well as practical tips on several aspects of a healthy lifestyle, weight loss, and physical activity. These are all great tools for getting support and meeting people who have goals similar to yours! Usually, users of internet health communities exchange social support by communicating via discussion forums, blogs, instant messaging and e-mail [115]. This allows you to experience social support regardless of your location, social circle or physical disability [116]. Furthermore, the option to post anonymous messages facilitates discussion of sensitive topics, while the diversity of online platforms means access to a vast network of peers from across the world, contributing to an enriching exchange of experiences. This expansion of your personal network may be particularly useful if you feel stigmatized by your current weight, or have limited mobility [117]. However, I strongly recommend some sort of online support for everyone. Why? Because online support works! When people are trying to lose weight, the use of internet-based programs with social support – including forums and communities – motivate them to persist in their efforts to lose weight thus they are more successful at losing and keeping the weight off [118]. However, while the internet is now a central part of many peoples' lives, face-to-face contact is still superior – so involve your spouse, best friend or colleague at work in your efforts, they may be just the help that enables you to lose weight and maintain your new, healthy body!

Successful Loser: Steve C.

Age: 29 years old

Weight lost: 62 pounds

Weight maintained for: 5 years

Steve C., a 29 years old lawyer who has lost 62 pounds, told me how he lost the weight and stayed skinny. "I gained my fair share of extra pounds when I went to college. All those changes leaving my parents' house to live in a student dorm – and the lifestyle that I had – partying, drinking, and my complete lack of cooking skills. It all added up, and I didn't really care." By the time Steve C. was in his senior year, he had gained more than 50 pounds! That was when he realized things could not continue as they were. "I made a deal with my roommate that both of us would graduate weighing the same as when we had started college. Since we are both very competitive, we agreed that whoever got to their pre-college weight first (and kept it for 6 months), would pay for a joint trip to Mexico. This really motivated us to keep going, because our pride was on the line and all of our friends knew about the bet. I started getting up at 5 am to run a couple of miles three times a week, and enrolled in a cooking class on campus to learn how to make healthy food. As it turns out, I was not the one who won the bet but I still managed to achieve my ideal weight with 2 months to spare. I lost the bet but won a great body!"

Tips from Successful losers:

❖ Successful Losers recognize the importance of their social network for achieving their goals. They choose their supporters carefully, and make sure that they are agreed on what role they are to play.

❖ If your significant other is getting between you and your goals, you need to talk to them to get them onboard. Explain to them what you are going through, and ask for their support. They may not even realize what they are doing wrong!

❖ Make sure that not only your supporters, but also all of the people close to you are informed about what you are planning. It also helps very much if they support your goals. Otherwise, your journey to losing weight will be a lot more difficult than it has to be.

❖ Social support is an important ally that can be found also online – regardless of whether you are trying to lose or maintain weight, or make other lifestyle changes. It can also be fun!

❖ There are many ways to get social support, so find one (or two) that suit your personality and lifestyle. That is what Successful Losers do.

[Secret X]

Recognize the challenge ahead

*"Our greatest glory is not in never falling, but in rising up
every time we fall."*

Ralph Waldo Emerson

Old habits die hard! Changing a habit is not an easy task, but rather requires a lot of effort from you. But the more you practice, the easier it gets! After achieving their goals, Successful Losers experience the joyful freedom and rewarding feelings of finally having accomplished what they have longed for, in many cases, their entire lives. Now that they are able to run a marathon, fit in a size 8 dress, and eat healthily on a daily basis – what comes next? I wish that I could tell you it is all over, that they live effortlessly happily ever after. But I would be lying! The maintenance of new and empowering habits must be a commitment for life. As you achieve your goals, you may feel like you have made it, that from now on you can relax and not worry about a thing. Big mistake! Nothing is as easy as falling back into old, comforting habits!

"Weight loss is a long-term venture that requires constant work, but that also offers continuous rewards"

As you have seen, Successful Losers are people just like you and me – but with more empowering thoughts and habits. Before becoming Successful Losers, they faced many of the challenges that you are facing now. They have cried, sweated, laughed, felt hopeless – just like you! However, they have continued on their journey to a healthy lifestyle. Sometimes, life does not go your way and you never know when that will happen. But regardless of what happens, Successful Losers know that they must keep their commitment to their new habits. Otherwise, none of the positive changes will last! Some Successful Losers even claim that once they had achieved their goals, they had to expend the same amount of effort on maintaining their new diet and activity levels – but without the positive experiences of seeing the weight drop, or being complimented by family and friends – who by now are used to the new ways [111]. So why bother?

Successful Losers and their "fat selves"

Even Successful Losers can regain weight if they do not continue to pursue the lifestyle that turned them into Successful Losers in the first place. Right now, it probably seems like a lot of work to maintain a healthy lifestyle forever, but the truth is that the more you practice a new habit, the more natural it becomes.

Successful Loser: Derek B.

Age: 37 years old

Weight lost: 60 pounds

Weight loss maintained for: 4 years

Derek B., a 37 years old library clerk, says: "Before I had achieved my goal of losing 60 pounds, everyone was very impressed by my discipline and hard work. But afterwards my efforts to keep the new weight were taken for granted. No one recognizes my ongoing efforts, or acknowledge that I still have to work very hard to keep my new body. I have to be careful not to become overconfident, or too complacent. You have to find the balance between knowing that you can do something, and still being conscious about the risk of possible setbacks and slip-ups."

However, in the end it is worth it! Not only because of the physical rewards such as climbing that flight of stairs without losing your breath, looking great in your old clothes, being healthy again, and playing effortlessly on the beach with your kids/nieces/dogs, but also because of the higher self-esteem, more active social life, and the feeling of accomplishment that comes with success.
Interviewing Successful Losers for this book, almost all claimed that their turning point came with the recognition that changes were needed that would last for a lifetime. They created a mindset where weight loss is a long-term venture that requires constant work, but that also offers continuous rewards. Successful Losers

report a conscious move away from a dieting mentality to a more relaxed approach where they do not worry about indulging in a few treats – but rather focus on changing their habits of everyday life. In fact, most said that they avoided explicitly banning any foods, as this had in the past led to feelings of being deprived while inevitably making the banned food more desirable. On the other hand, food and weight maintenance are two things that are always on Successful Losers' minds, and they all had an established set of rules or boundaries regarding eating that they lived by. They constantly evaluate what they "can and cannot get away with", especially in the weight maintenance phase. To this end, they use written records a lot. Successful Losers also described being more in touch with their bodies and having a greater understanding of their nutritional needs and food desires. They listen to their bodies more, and also question whether they really want a particular food. Because their daily life is under control, they can sometimes indulge their whims!

Furthermore, Successful Losers accept that lapses are a part of life, and when they happen they are prepared to quickly move on back to their healthy routines rather than dwelling on each lapse. All Successful Losers know that their success depends on balanced, regular and planned meals containing healthy food. They report that the most effective strategy to healthy eating is to reduce sweets, processed foods and alcohol.

A great example of a Successful Loser who faced her demons to find the secret for a healthy and happy life based on choice is Helen J.

Successful Loser: Helen J.

Age: 49 years old

Weight lost: 104 pounds

Weight loss maintained for: 11 years

Helen J., 49, has lost a stunning 104 pounds – and maintained her new weight for more than ten years. She says: "I don't know how many times I tried to lose weight; I have bought into everything modern medicine can offer – from starvation diets to weight-loss surgery. But I always ended up gaining the weight back. Do you know how humiliating it is to go through weight-loss surgery and still remain fat? I do, and I will never forget the feeling of being a complete failure. After this episode, I suddenly realized that I and no one else had to take charge of the situation! I figured out that I must change my attitude towards life. Eating healthily could no longer be the same as being on a diet. I decided that living and eating healthily would be part of my life for as long as I live. No more periods of starvation followed by weeks or months of binge eating. I promised myself that I would only cultivate habits that I could keep for a lifetime, and that made me feel more relaxed towards the whole thing. I have always been very much focused on results, but never really realized that results in life only matter if the journey to get there is possible and pleasant. I know that I have lost a lot of weight and that I am in control of my life – but I also know that the only way to keep slim is to be consistent in my healthy lifestyle. Those habits made me a Successful Loser."

Biologically, the human body is designed to be in balance. If you burn more calories than you eat you will lose weight, but if you eat more than you need the extra calories are stored as fat. Once your fat cells are formed, you can never get rid of them – and when they die new ones come to replace them. Fat cells are mostly formed during childhood, which is why it is more difficult to lose weight and stay slim for those of us who have been overweight or obese in childhood. When you do lose weight, your fat cells shrink – but do not disappear. They are just sitting there like empty fuel tanks, waiting for you to have an excess of calories again – which is when you gain weight and your fat cells grow again in order to store all that new fat. Eat too much and new fat cells may even be created. During your entire life, your fat cells grow or shrink depending on the amount of calories you routinely eat [119]. So even if you were obese as a child and have a lot of fat cells, you are not predestined to be fat. Experts agree that the most important determinants of body fat and obesity are all related to modifiable lifestyle factors – such as your diet and physical activity habits.

This is why I would like to introduce you to your evil twin – your "fat self". In addition to our biological drive to make sure that we eat enough and store excess energy as fat in the body, there is what I like to call the "fat self". The "fat self" is that part of your brain that is always urging you to take the easy way out, that tries to convince you that you don't really need to be physically active, that unconsciously looks at the slices of cake on offer and always attempts to get the bigger one, and the one that keeps you eating even when you are no longer hungry. This "fat self" loves nothing more than to devour a big portion of ice-cream in front of the TV, feels pure joy when the delivery man knocks on your door with a four-cheese pizza and urges you to forget about tomorrow and eat today! It makes you rely on emotional eating when you face difficulties in life, and it is always on the lookout for any excuse not to go to the gym. Do you recognize your "fat self" now? Let me also tell you that it is something that you have inherited from your stone age forebears, but that is no longer useful. It may even harm you! In fact, as we have heard, even after losing weight the Successful Losers have to keep watching out for their "fat selves". However, they know that this part of their brain will always be there. To permanently lose weight, they just have to work around it, realizing that it is not relevant in today's world of plenty. In fact, many of the secrets are ways to specifically silence your "fat self" in daily life – now you try it!

Tips from Successful losers:

❖ Successful Losers are as human as you are. If they made it, so can you!

❖ Successful Losers know that their continued success is due to their constant focus on maintaining a healthy lifestyle – the habits that turned them into Successful Losers in the first place.

❖ No pain, no gain! Successful Losers know that to get what they want, they will have to go through some short-term pain. But they also know that in the long-term the gains are worth it. What about you?

❖ Learn to recognize when your "fat self" is calling the shots – then show it who the boss is!

❖ Achieving your goals is fantastic, but keeping on achieving them is even better!

Part III

Tricks of the trade – What do expert dietitians know that you don't?

[6]

Why calories matter

If you are living on planet Earth, you have probably heard the word calorie. Ah, you say, the infamous calories! Commonly best avoided as an enemy and feared by all trying to lose weight. But is this reputation for danger really well deserved, or is it just a widespread misunderstanding? By definition, a calorie is the amount of energy that raises the temperature of 1 gram (or 0.03 oz) of water by 1 degree Celsius (or 1.8 Fahrenheit). The key word here is energy. Calories are energy. And energy is also what fuels your body and keeps you alive, warm and able to function! If deprived of enough calories, your heart would stop, your lungs would not draw breath, and your brain would shut down. In other words, you would die. So we need calories, just not too many of them! But how do you know how many calories your body needs to keep healthy and well?

The truth is there is no single answer that fits all bodies. Both because the calories in the food that you eat are converted into energy slightly differently, and because the energy that is generated is used by your body in different ways depending on your physical activity level, stress and indeed your overall health. Each one of us has a basic (but personal) calorie need just to keep living – some of it because of the way you are built, the rest depending on your gender, age, physical activity level, body weight and amount of muscle. In general, an adult needs at least 1000 to 1400 calories daily to have enough energy to fuel key organs like the brain, heart, and lungs. Even if you do not move at all, you still need to attain this minimum caloric intake to guarantee your vital functions. This minimum number of calories is called the resting metabolic rate.

> *"Calories are energy. And energy is also what fuels your*
> *body and keeps you alive, warm and able to function!"*

On top of this, in order to have enough energy to be active, we all need extra energy typically amounting to about 400 to 600 additional calories per day, but varying widely depending on physical activity and if you want to lose, maintain or gain weight. Yes, there are some people who actually want to gain weight! In the table below there are the estimated calories recommende d for maintaining weight in typical adult women and men [120]. However, remember that these are estimates that may or may not work for you!

In general, men need more energy to fuel their bodies than women, as men typically have bigger and more muscular bodies. And more, due to reductions in resting metabolic rate that occur with aging, calorie needs generally decrease with age. If you are not sure how physically active you are, read on to find out the answer!

Physical activity level

Gender	Age	Sedentary	Moderately active	Active
Women	19 - 30	1800 -2000 kcal	2000 -2200 kcal	2400 kcal
	31 - 50	1800 kcal	2000 kcal	2200 kcal
	51+	1600 kcal	1800 kcal	2000 - 2200 kcal

Gender	Age	Sedentary	Moderately active	Active
Men	19 - 30	2400 – 2600 kcal	2600 - 2800 kcal	3000 kcal
	31 - 50	2200 – 2400 kcal	2400 – 2600 kcal	2800 – 3000 kcal
	51+	2000 – 2200 kcal	2200 – 2400 kcal	2400 – 2800 kcal

How physically active are you?

Most of us like to think that we are more physically active than we really are and that we eat less than we really do. There is nothing wrong in being optimistic, but the problem is that you may never achieve your goals if you do not have a factual understanding of how physically active you actually are. Also, remember our previous discussion on differences between exercise and physical activity. When it comes to physical activity, most people fall into one of these categories:

Sedentary – If this is you, your lifestyle includes only the light physical activity associated with typical day-to-day life. For example, you work in an office or have other sedentary work, and when you are at home you spend most of your time sitting down watching TV, playing video games or reading. You may walk up the occasional stair, but you never walk more than one mile in any one day.

Moderately active – If this is you, your daily life includes more than the light physical activity associated with typical day-to-day life. To qualify, you also have to do the equivalent of walking 1.5 miles per day, or practicing a sport (including going to the gym) at least three times a week. Alternatively, you may work in an environment that demands moderate daily physical activity, such as waiting on tables or delivering goods.

Active – If this is you, congratulations! Your lifestyle not only includes the light physical activity associated with day-to-day life, but also additional physical activity equivalent to walking more than 3 miles daily, or practicing a sport (including going to the gym) five or more times a week. Alternatively, you work in a very physically demanding job, for example as an aerobics instructor or manual construction worker [121].

How active should you be?

Getting adequate amounts of physical activity is one of the best medicines known, and confers many additional health benefits regardless of body weight. Regular participation in physical activity helps you to maintain a healthy weight, and prevents weight gain. Furthermore, physical activity, particularly when combined with a reduced calorie intake, aids weight loss and the maintenance of weight loss – just ask any Successful Loser!

The amount of physical activity necessary to successfully maintain a healthy body weight depends on your basal metabolic rate and your calorie intake, and varies considerably. To achieve the amounts of physical activity recommended to maintain good health, you should do the equivalent of 150 minutes of moderate-intensity aerobic (movements that leave you short of breath) activity each week [121] – these should be divided into several weekly sessions, for example 50 minutes of physical activity three times a week or 30 minutes five days a week. However, if you are sedentary these numbers may discourage you from even starting as it might be more than you think you can handle. My advice for you is to start moving as much as you can anyway – even if you do not reach the minimum recommended. As you become more fit, then you should gradually increase the amount of time spent on physical activity.

If you want to lose weight, you should increase your weekly minutes of physical activity gradually over time while at the same time slowly decreasing your calorie intake to a point where you start losing about 0.5 to 1 pounds per week. Then, keep the same calorie intake while continuing to increase the amount of physical activity to reach a healthy weight. Remember, you may need a higher/lower level of physical activity than others to achieve and maintain a healthy body weight. That is why it is so important to find out what works for you!

Using calories to lose weight

A typical recommended daily calorie intake to maintain your current weight should be adjusted for your gender, age and physical activity level. If you want to lose weight over time, you should consume about 500 calories less than the minimum indicated for you. To lose weight, you will need to convince your body to burn more calories than you consume. However, this is a process that begins with energy from your muscles, then from your liver and finally (after about 2-4 days) from your fat stores. Simply put, it is an unbreakable law of nature that if you consume more calories than you use, you gain weight as the extra calories are stored for later use, while if you consume fewer calories than your body needs over time you will lose weight. However, starve yourself too much and you will not be able to maintain normal body functions, and soon you will start to break down essential body parts (such as muscles) just to fuel your breathing! Finally, if you have a balance between energy intake and energy expenditure, you will maintain your current weight. As simple as that!

Going back to the dieting subject, it is important to remember that drastically reducing your calorie intake for a short period of time may seem to be a quick and easy way to lose weight, but it is actually not. This is because your body can rarely continue a very restrictive diet for long, especially if you are eating fewer calories than necessary to keep up with your resting metabolic rate. Realizing the danger of running out of fuel long before your fat has melted away, your body will make sure that you eat whatever and whenever you can! If you are dieting right now, I can guarantee that you will fail to keep your weight loss in the long term if you do not change your lifestyle. Why don't you stop this harmful practice and instead start applying the Successful Losers' lifestyle secrets for losing weight and keeping it off? Chances are that you already know how bad starvation feels, and how easy it is to eventually make up for those missing calories by overeating and gaining back the weight lost. But that is not all; your body is deprived of its necessary fuel suddenly and dramatically when you diet. Besides sending out distressed hunger signals, it will also cause your resting metabolic rate to decrease, meaning that you now have to consume even less calories to continue to lose weight! Successful Losers know this, which is why they never diet.

How are calories related to fat and muscle?

We have seen that if you consume more calories than your body requires each day, you will eventually gain weight. And most of this weight is gained as fat, because fat is a great store of energy. In a small volume, it can store a lot of energy. It is stable, easy to maintain and also functions as insulation. Amazingly, it takes an accumulated excess of 3500 calories to gain just 1 pound of fat! If your body needs 1600 calories a day to maintain its current weight, while you consume 2100 (one 4 oz chocolate chip muffin extra, or about 500 calories), you would have to keep going for exactly one week to add 1 pound of body fat. Likewise, if you are eating 2000 calories a day and maintaining your weight, you would need to burn 250 calories (one hour of brisk walking) per day to lose 0.5 pounds of fat in one week. If you also cut down your caloric intake by 250 calories a day (a 2 oz Milky Way bar), resulting in the larger deficit of 500 calories a day, you could easily lose 1 pound of fat per week.

Muscle, on the other hand, requires a lot of energy to maintain so is not very efficient for storing excess energy, as well as being a source of heat loss rather than insulation. In other words, the more muscle you have in your body, the more calories (energy) you will need to consume to make it work. Successful Losers know that muscles are their friend, which is why they usually add weight training to their fitness routines.

Now that you know how physically active you are, what calories are and how you may lose, gain or keep your weight using them, it is time to find out where calories come from and why you should eat food from all of the nutrient groups – as you can guess, in moderation.

Chapter 6 in a nutshell

❖ Calories are nothing more than energy! And energy is what our bodies need to survive – just not too much of it!

❖ Your calorie needs are directly related to your calorie expenditure, so the more calories (energy) that you burn, the more calories you are able to eat without gaining weight.

❖ Because caloric foods are tasty foods, Successful Losers generally have a moderately to very active lifestyle – which means that they can enjoy the occasional treat. What about you?

❖ Aim for at least 150 minutes of physical activity per week – that is 50 minutes three times a week or 30 minutes five times a week.

❖ Dieting stresses your body and causes it to slow down your basal metabolic rate, making it much more difficult for you to burn calories and lose weight – which is why Successful Losers never diet!

[7]

Not all foods are created equal

We all need food to live. Eating is the most important need after breathing and drinking (water that is!). As we have seen throughout this book, without food there is no life. By now, you also know through experience how important food is to life and happiness – but do you know what your food is made of? What kind of nutritional benefits are you getting from the food you eat? And what should you be eating to achieve your goals? If your answer to any of these questions is no, then this chapter is for you.

By definition, food is any substance consumed to provide nutritional support for our bodies [122]. It is usually of plant or animal origin, and contains at least some macronutrients (such as carbohydrates, fats, proteins) and micronutrients (vitamins and minerals) [122]. Successful Losers know that to maintain a healthy weight, they need to rely on a wide variety of foods to get the job done – but also the knowledge of these foods and how they affect the body is key. So, let start with a crash course in nutrition!

What are macronutrients and what are they for?

Macronutrients are nutrients that contain calories. Basically, they are grouped into carbohydrates, proteins and fats – alcohol also contains calories but it is not considered a macronutrient as it does not provide any benefits beside energy and has a lot of side effects. Each macronutrient has its own specific functions and also interacts with the other macronutrients to build our bodies. A healthy and balanced diet should always contain at least some carbohydrates, some protein, and – yes – some fat. To manage your weight, you should consume a diet that has an appropriate number of calories, and that provides adequate amounts of each macronutrient as well as plenty of vitamins and minerals. There is no optimal proportion of macronutrients that facilitates weight loss or helps with maintaining weight loss.

"A healthy diet consists of carbohydrates, proteins, and fats"

Although some well-known diets promote the consumption of one macronutrient (such as protein) over the others, and although some of these diets temporarily work, more important than the relative distribution of macronutrients in the diet is whether or not the diet is low in calories, easily maintained over time and prevents your body from experiencing constant hunger [120]. Indeed, in the nutrition field, it is agreed that the total number of calories consumed sustainably over time is more important than the proportion of carbohydrates, proteins and fats in your diet when it comes to lose weight [120].

Based on the above and on my own experience, as well as on the eating habits of Successful Losers, the best current dietary advice for those attempting weight loss and/or weight maintenance is to choose a balanced diet with adequate macronutrients (carbohydrates, proteins and fats), a number of calories suited to your energy needs, and especially one that agrees with you – you will be eating like this for a long, long time! If you are unsure, I recommend a low-fat, high-carbohydrate diet with a high fiber content [123], which will keep you full for longer and is easy to obtain in both restaurants and supermarkets.

Carbohydrates – good or bad?

Recently, carbohydrates have gained a reputation as saboteurs of diets. This reputation has been propagated by various media outlets – from serious scientific journals, TV shows, and popular diet books to tabloid papers worldwide. As a nutrition expert, I am constantly asked by people from every walk of life if they can or should eat carbohydrates. These questions usually vary from: "Is it true that carbs can make me fat?" or "I love pasta, but I hear that it is not good for me" to "I know someone who lost a lot of weight by eating protein and fat – is that good?" Unfortunately, only part of the carbohydrates story ever makes it into the media! The other half you will learn in this chapter! Let's start from the beginning. What are carbohydrates and what are they for?

Carbohydrates are our bodies' main source of energy! Each 0.03 oz (1 gram) of carbohydrate provides 4 kcal, and this energy is used to make glucose – which is the fuel that keeps your body going, including your muscles and your brain. Unlike other nutrients that need to be processed to be of use, your body can burn glucose immediately, or choose to store it in your liver and muscles for when it is needed. However, eat too much carbohydrates and the excess is stored as fat to be used during a coming starvation (that will likely never happen) [124].

Nonetheless, carbohydrates in the right amounts are a healthy and important part of your diet, but as everything else they should be consumed in moderation. It is also good to know that there are two groups of carbohydrates: simple carbs (sometimes called fast carbs), including sugars, and complex carbs (sometimes called slow carbs), including starches and fibers.

The so-called simple carbohydrates are like glucose very easily accessible as sources of energy for the body, and mostly come from highly processed foods that in the process lose much of their vitamin and nutrient content. Simple carbs are easily transformed by the body into glucose – elevating your blood sugar levels which may over time make you prone to be fat and can trigger latent type-2 diabetes. Complex carbs, as their name suggests, have a more complex natural chemistry that makes them harder for the body to burn immediately or to convert into glucose. Complex carbs mostly come directly from nature, without much processing, and as a consequence they are often rich in nutrients such as iron, magnesium, selenium, B vitamins and dietary fiber. Whole grains are a good source of complex carbs, although they vary in their dietary fiber content. In fact, eating whole grain regularly may reduce your risk of cardiovascular disease, and is associated with a lower body weight.

Simple vs. Complex Carbs: who wins?

As we have seen, carbohydrates are a central part of our modern diets, and are found in everything from fruits and vegetables (mostly complex), breads and cereals (both), to other grains (mostly complex), milk and milk products (simple), and sweet foods (e.g., cakes, cookies, and sugar-sweetened beverages like soda – all made mostly with simple carbs) [124]. While some simple carbs are found naturally in foods (such as lactose in milk and fructose in fruit), most are added (such as table sugar added to muffins and high fructose corn syrup in sugar-sweetened beverages).

Similarly, complex carbs are often naturally occurring (such as in beans and whole grains), but are also often added (fiber-enriched breakfast cereal, whole grain bread) [120]. To further complicate things, most carbohydrates are consumed in the form of starches, which may be either simple or complex. Starches are found in foods such as grains, potatoes, and refined grains like pasta – remember to check the label. Most people today consume an adequate (or too high) amount of total carbohydrates, but mostly in the form of simple carbs and not complex carbs, especially fiber, which is the really healthy kind of carb [120].

In fact, the majority of sugar in the typical American diet is added during processing, preparation, or at the table. These "added sugars" (invariably simple carbs) sweeten the flavor of foods and beverages to improve their taste. They are also added for preservation purposes (too much sugar makes it hard for many bacteria to thrive!) and to provide functional attributes, such as texture, body, and color.

Whole grains – the super carbs

Whole grains – defied as grains that retain their outer casing, or bran – differ from refined grains in that the latter only retain the inner energy supply (called endosperm). Whole grains are a key source of micronutrients such as iron, magnesium, selenium and B vitamins, as well as of dietary fiber. Dietary fiber is actually something that naturally occurs in plants where it provides structure and form, but when it is eaten it helps to provide a feeling of fullness and keeps your intestines healthy by keeping them busy. As it is expected, whole grains vary in their dietary fiber content, with some of the best sources of dietary fiber found among beans and peas, including navy beans, split peas, lentils, pinto beans, and black beans. Other sources of dietary fiber also play a role in a healthy diet, including vegetables, fruits, and nuts. The current dietary recommendation for fiber is 25 g per day for women and 38 g per day for men – most of us eat far less than that. To lose weight and stay healthy, you should aim to replace many refined-grain foods (simple carbs) with whole-grain foods (complex carbs). Use the nutritional facts label to help you, as already discussed in Secret VIII. It is probably unrealistic for most of us to only eat unrefined grains, so when you eat refined grains try to make sure that they are enriched with vitamins, minerals and fiber. But for the most part, if you want to eat healthily and lose weight, you must eat complex carbs, and most of those in the form of whole grains.

The take home message is that eating a lot of carbohydrates can actually be healthy, as long as they are complex carbohydrates. In fact, this diet is not only more nutritious and lower in calories, it also provides enough fuel for your busy lifestyle – and it is similar to what our ancestors ate (and thus what we were built to eat)!

Proteins – the building blocks of life

Like carbohydrates, proteins also provide 4 kcal per 0.03 oz (1 gram). Additionally, unlike carbs, proteins provide the amino acids that are the main building blocks of your body's tissues. Amino acids are either essential or non-essential, with essential amino acids being, well, essential because the body can't manufacture them by itself – they must be obtained from our diet. Consequently, your diet should provide enough protein to provide enough essential amino acids [125]. Luckily, proteins are found in a wide variety of both animal and plant foods. Animal-based protein foods include seafood, meat, poultry, eggs, milk and milk products – these protein sources are usually called complete because they provide all the different amino acids. Most plant sources of proteins are considered incomplete because of their low content of one or more of the essential amino acids – more about that below [125].

Both plant and animal-based sources of proteins can be equally well incorporated into a healthy eating pattern. However, some animal-based protein sources are high in saturated fat, so low-fat choices should be selected – if you want to eat mainly animal protein [120, 125]. If you prefer a vegetarian diet, you can still get the right amounts of protein but you need to learn how to combine different types of plant sources of protein to get all of the essential amino acids your body needs. For example, mixing rice with beans is a great choice as they complement each other's amino acid composition.

A study of attempted weight loss in 90 overweight and obese women looked at the importance of protein and calcium content in the diet as part of a program also featuring regular exercise. All participants were able to lose weight (and fat); however, those participants who consumed a high protein and calcium diet lost more weight than the others [126]. Why? Well, the participants who ate more protein also gained more muscle – which as we have seen in Chapter 6 helps to burn fat and maintain weight loss, also when you are not exercising. The researchers concluded that a planned diet combined with regular exercise can induce weight loss, especially when combined with high levels of protein and calcium to promote increased muscle mass.

If you are wondering how much protein you need each day, the current recommendation is that 10–35% of your daily calories should come from protein. For a standard diet, that comes out to around 46 grams a day for women and 56 grams a day for men [125].

Fats – What are they for?

Dietary fats have an undeservedly bad reputation! They add taste, consistence, flavor, energy and make you feel full longer after eating. Dietary fats come in many varieties, and are found in both plant and animal foods. Because 0.03 oz (or 1 gram) of fat contains 9 kcal, along with essential fatty acids and the fat-soluble vitamins A, D, E, and K, even a little fat contains a lot of energy – which is why you store energy as fat in the first place. There are established ranges for total fat intake for adults (ages 19 years and older: 20–35%). These ranges are based on the reduced risk of many chronic diseases, such as cardiovascular disease, when keeping below the higher threshold, while keeping above the lower threshold means getting an adequate intake of essential nutrients.

Even with the high calorie content of fat, those of us who are trying to lose weight can still eat fat – but the amount and type of fat in the diet should be managed wisely to control total energy intake [123]. Most people consume more than enough fat (especially the bad types of fat – saturated and trans fats), but usually not enough of the good type of fat (monounsaturated and polyunsaturated fats).

The facts about fat

The good: Monounsaturated and polyunsaturated fats

The "good" types of fat are considered good because they reduce overall cholesterol levels, and specifically help to decrease "bad" cholesterol associated with heart disease while boosting the "good" cholesterol that is linked to improved cardiovascular health. These fats are also known as monounsaturated and polyunsaturated fats and are found in seafood, nuts, seeds, and vegetable oils, amongst other sources. The "good" fats should replace the "bad" and the "evil" fats (more on these below) as often as possible, especially in your frying pan or wok! However, even if they are "good", these fats should be eaten in moderation. Remember, they are still fats – and each 0.03 oz still contains 9 kcal! In my experience, the "good" fats are best used to replace the "bad" fats in dishes that call for added fat. For example, you can replace some fatty meats (like burgers) and poultry (like chicken wings) with seafood or skinless chicken breast, and use vegetable oils instead of solid fats such as butter in all of your cooking. If you eat a lot of dairy products, you can also try replacing them with healthier alternatives made from soya or oat – or just use the non-fat versions.

The bad: Saturated fats and cholesterol

Your body needs very small amounts of saturated fat to function, but it makes this fat by itself when it is needed. Therefore, you have no dietary requirement for saturated fat. In addition, a high intake of saturated fat is associated with higher levels of total cholesterol, especially the "bad" cholesterol, atherosclerosis and other risk factors for heart disease. Also, consuming less than 10 percent of the calories you need in the form of saturated fat – replacing the rest with "good" fat – helps to lower blood cholesterol levels and a reduce the risk of heart disease.

Even though there are many kinds of cholesterol particles in the blood, they are generally divided into "good" cholesterol (as fat storage to be used as energy) and "bad" cholesterol (fat going the other way – to be stored or even built into your arteries as atherosclerosis). When it comes to cholesterol, you should eat as little as possible since your body produces all you need on its own. In your diet, cholesterol is found only in animal foods, especially eggs, chicken, beef, and all types of sausages and hamburgers.

The evil: Trans fats

Trans fats are a special kind of fat that is resistant to aging, helping to conserve foods for longer. While small amounts of trans fats can be found naturally in some foods, they are much more common as manufactured additives to processed foods such as cookies, cakes, potato chips, crackers, fried foods and most fast-food. A number of studies have observed an association between a high trans fat intake and an increased risk of heart disease and death. This increased risk is at least partly due to a rise in "bad" cholesterol and a decrease in "good" cholesterol that occurs when eating trans fats [127]. With no benefits and a lot of risks, we all have good reason to avoid trans fats as much as possible.

Micronutrients – vitamins and minerals

Vitamins are organic substances (made by plants or animals), while minerals are inorganic elements that come from the earth (but may be absorbed by plants and eaten that way). Animals and humans mostly absorb minerals from the fruits and plants they eat. Vitamins and minerals are together called micronutrients – important nutrients that our body needs to grow and develop normally but that are only needed in small quantities and that do not add any energy (calories) to our diets. Vitamins may be essential (not possible for the body to make on its own) or non-essential (made by the body as needed) and often help the body to function by facilitating certain reactions. Most minerals are needed in very small doses, and because of that they are called trace minerals. Examples are chromium, copper, iodine, iron, selenium, and zinc. Despite being much less abundant than the macronutrients, vitamins and minerals play a unique role in maintaining our health. For example, vitamin D helps our body absorb calcium (a mineral) needed to form strong bones and teeth. A deficiency in vitamin D can result in a disease called rickets (softening of the bones caused by an inability to absorb enough calcium). The best way to get enough micronutrients is to eat a balanced diet with a variety of foods, especially from the plant kingdom. You usually get all the micronutrients that you need from the foods you eat [128] – unless you are on a starvation-type diet or a very picky eater.

Bad food or just the wrong amounts?

As we have seen in this chapter, there is no such thing as good or bad food. Even the healthiest foods can make you fat if you eat too much of them. In fact, I remember a funny story that a professor in an undergraduate nutrition course told a class several years ago. One of her patients who desperately wanted to lose weight was informed that she should eat one, and only one, fruit before each meal to feel less hungry and therefore eat less. The exact type of fruit was not specified. After 4 weeks, this patient returned to the clinic for a follow-up consultation. Surprisingly, she had gained 5 pounds. When asked what she had been eating during the time at home, the patient swore that she had followed the diet plan perfectly. She reported proudly that she "indeed ate one whole fruit before each and every meal throughout, not missing a single one! But I have to tell you that it was tough going getting through three mangos every day – and on top of my usual meals"!

My point in telling you this story is that all calories may not be created the same, but if they are consumed in excess even healthy calories will make you fat – just as eating small portions of so-called unhealthy foods will not automatically make you fat. It has been scientifically proven that some highly caloric foods – such as dark chocolate, wine and vegetable oils (monounsaturated and polyunsaturated fats) – can actually contribute to health and even weight loss if eaten in small amounts. Since these foods provide healthy nutrients and keep you full for longer, they help you to avoiding unhealthy snacks and overeating. This is why it's not such a bad idea to keep such items on your menu!

Indeed, not all foods are created equal and some can even turn you into a food addict. In the next chapter, you will learn about the physiology of food addiction and how to break free from this malady.

Chapter 7 in a nutshell

❖ All macronutrients (carbohydrates, proteins and fats) and micronutrients (vitamins and minerals) are essential parts of a healthy and balanced diet.

❖ Carbohydrates are not the obesogenic substance that many fad diets want you to believe. But make sure that you eat mostly complex carbs while avoiding as much as possible simple carbs that unleash a wave of (probably not needed) energy on your body.

❖ Proteins are the building blocks of life! To get all the nutritional benefits minus the harmful fats, choose lean sources of protein.

❖ Fats are good! As long as you eat mostly the healthy kinds (monounsaturated and polyunsaturated) but avoid the bad (saturated fat and cholesterol) and completely abstain from the evil (trans) kinds of fat.

❖ There is no such thing as good or bad food. Even the healthiest foods can make you fat if you eat too much of them.

[8]

Food is more than nutrition – it is a drug!

Are you addicted to food? Actually, hunger is one of the most powerful urges there is, and eating triggers a blissful sensation like no other – which is logical if you think about what would happen should we neglect to eat for a while! Eating is not only refilling our energy balance and then being full; it is also a pleasure and a reward. As we have seen previously in this book, your eating habits are dependent on so many other things than plain old hunger. What you eat reflects who you are and who you become, builds your character or destroys it, and can make you stronger and healthier or weaker and sick. But how can something so basic to survival be so harmful?

There is no such thing as completely good or entirely bad food. However, some foods when eaten in sufficient quantity can become addictive – turning you into a "food addict". These foods imprison you and make you a slave if you do not restrict your consumption. Such foods are usually processed foods rich in sugar, fat and salt. They are maliciously designed to make you want more, and are usually cheap, convenient and tasty. The more you eat them, the more you will want to eat. Worse, they make healthy food seem tasteless and unattractive. If it were not for their negative consequences for your health and lifespan, these foods would be perfect!

*"Some foods when eaten in sufficient quantity can
become addictive – turning you into a food addict"*

In my experience, it is more and more common to hear people say that they are addicted to some types of food. Usually, the term "addiction" implies psychological and physical dependence on a substance – including alcohol, tobacco, heroin or other drugs which temporarily alter the chemical balance in the brain [129]. When a person is addicted, or "dependent", on a drug they become compulsive – sometimes uncontrollable – in behaviors aimed at obtaining the drug and its effects, which they are ready to prioritize over other actions more important for a long and happy life [13]. Chronic overeaters report going through a similar process – compulsively planning or working on obtaining the next (usually sweet and fatty) meal.

Like addicts of other drugs, food addicts describe symptoms of withdrawal when they are deprived of their favorite foods.

Another aspect of food addiction is food cravings, usually involving sugary foods – such as chocolate, candy and ice cream. These foods trigger feelings of well-being and impulsive eating in all of us, but much more strongly in food addicts [13]. So, like most addictions, the food addict starts small with perhaps a favorite sugary food, but loses control and ends up in a vicious cycle of self-indulgence that may result in obesity or an eating disorder

Not surprisingly, tasty foods activate the brain's reward system, relying on mechanisms similar to those triggered by alcohol and nicotine. Because of this powerful kick, the addict feels an uncontrollable need to eat certain foods [130]. Sometimes you may feel powerless when confronted with a highly appealing food that stimulates your appetite, even when you are not hungry. Unfortunately, our brain biology for appetite regulation has not been constructed for today's high exposure to tasty food [13]!

How sugar works in your brain

Have you ever felt the excitement of a sugar high? If so, you know that soon after the buzz comes the crash! Sugar is the brain's main source of energy - but when it comes in the wrong form (read simple carbs), it may instead disrupt the brain's finely tuned appetite control. If you consistently eat foods rich in simple sugars you will experience big swings in your blood sugar levels. And when your blood sugar is low, you will instinctively crave another dose of sugar to make you feel good again. The next thing you know, you are stuck in the vicious cycle of sugar addiction!

These observations from my clinical practice have a basis in science. Several regions of the brain that are involved in initiating feeding behavior are also involved in drug abuse [131, 132]. In an in-depth review of the literature, researchers from Princeton University concluded that "food is not ordinarily like a substance of abuse, but alternating bingeing and deprivation changes that. Based on the observed behavioral and neurochemical similarities between the effects of sugar consumption and drug abuse, sugar, as common as it is, nonetheless meets the criteria for substance abuse and may be addictive for some individuals when consumed in a binge-like manner" [13]. Simple translation: sugar can be a drug if you abuse it! And because the negative effects of sugar take decades to appear, and because sugar is so common in our daily life, you may not even notice your addiction until it is too late. The drastic comparison between sugar and drugs actually comes from studies showing that the changes in brain chemistry that take place are similar for drugs and for sugar [13]. The good news is that sugar addiction is much weaker than being addicted to, say, alcohol or cocaine – meaning that it is easier to kick your food addiction than many others. Who would have guessed that such a commonly used substance can have such an addictive effect!

Do some people crave food more than others?

It seems that some people are unable to resist to food, while others must almost be reminded to eat – and that these differences are the result of more than just lacking self-control. Again, scientists have an answer. They have analyzed how slim and fat people respond to rewards that you can eat (like candy) and those that you can't (like money) [133, 134]. While everyone in the study agreed that money was a better reward than candy, overweight participants changed their behavior almost as much to get candy as to get money. Slim participants were not willing to work at all as hard. In fact, the more overweight you are, the harder you are willing to work for food. Why? Well, research is ongoing, but one explanation may be that when we become overweight, our brain's reward response to food is delayed, making us eat more than we should in order to feel a "sugar rush" [135].

Public enemy number one

If you cannot resist sweets, you are not alone! Americans of all ages and ethnicities are consuming more and more sugar – and we are not talking about slow-burning carbs! Simultaneously, we are in the middle of an epidemic of obesity, which in turn is connected to rapidly rising rates of diabetes, heart disease and may even be an important cause for why we now may be the first generation to live shorter lives than our parents [136]. Of the hundreds of studies linking overweight to sugar in the diet, few if any are accessible to the general reader. So you have to trust me when I say that there is a strong connection between the amounts of glucose and fructose (two different types of sugar) in the diet and obesity [137-139]. This is why states such as New York and California have considered taxing soft drinks!

Of glucose and fructose, I think that you know more about the first than about the second. But if you are serious about living healthily, you now need to read up on both of them! Fructose, also known as fruit sugar, is commonly found in foods and beverages – both occurring naturally (in fruits and juices) and as an added ingredient (such as in soft drinks, sweetened cereals, and pastries). Because of its many sources, fructose is not always labeled as such – in fact, the food label more commonly lists sucrose (table sugar, which contains equal amounts of glucose and fructose) or high fructose corn syrup (a common and inexpensive sweetener added to many food products). Excessive intake of fructose (>50 g/day) is linked to development of one of our most dangerous killers: the metabolic syndrome (obesity, hypertension, insulin resistance, and a high blood cholesterol) [140].

Fructose is a common, and therefore cheap, sweetener that is added to a vast range of foods (even those where you see no earthly reason for why it should be in there), but it has dangerous metabolic effects on the body when consumed in excess. Remember, our ancestors' diet did not contain much fructose – except for the occasional honeycomb or fruit. One of the many tricky things with fructose is that it is absorbed in the intestine like glucose (and sucrose, our regular table sugar), but does not stimulate the pancreas to release insulin like the other carbs [141-143]. Why? No one knows – but I do know that a healthy insulin response is important for food intake because high levels inhibit overeating [144] and increase the release of the satiety hormone leptin [145]. So instead of a high insulin response, which lowers blood glucose to healthy levels, fructose reduces the insulin response to sugar [146]! Even worse, fructose contains as many calories per oz as does glucose. So however much fructose you eat, you will never feel as full as after a meal that contains mostly other types of sugars (glucose or sucrose).

Because of import tariffs on sucrose and subsidies to corn farmers, we are figuratively drowning in fructose, in the form of high-fructose corn syrup. High-fructose corn syrup is cheap, tastes great and has unfortunately become a staple ingredient in our food [147]. Fructose can make you fat not only through tricking your appetite regulation, but also by adding a whole lot of extra calories [148] – a soda anyone? To make matter worse, the more fructose you eat, the less sensitive your brain becomes, and because of that you need to eat ever more sugar to get that rush – the next thing you know, you are stuck in a vicious cycle!

Today Americans consume nearly three times as much fructose per person and year as we did a century ago [148]. This is not only the fault of cheap and abundant high-fructose corn syrup, but also due to an increase in industrialized foods and a shift in consumer tastes to prefer sweet food. But since the 1960s, high-fructose corn syrup – super sweet and super cheap – has been helping manufacturers give us what we want. Amazingly, today soft drinks and other sugar-sweetened beverages are the main source of added sugars in the diet for most Americans [149]. That is why it is so important to avoid these drinks if you wish to restrict your added sugar intake – and become a Successful Loser.

What do Successful Losers do?

As they say, the difference between poison and medicine is the dose. A smart way to deal with cravings is to add small doses of healthy sweets to your diet instead of removing them completely. Successful Losers embrace healthy foods, but do not necessarily ban the foods they crave. Ironically, once you give your body what it wants in small doses, the cravings for huge portions disappear. Successful Losers control their food cravings by eating regularly (it is much easier to succumb to food cravings when you are hungry), drinking plenty of water, keeping healthy snacks on hand for when a craving pops up, and, most importantly, drastically reduce their intake of added or artificial sugars (the more you eat of these kinds of foods, the more you will want!). By maintaining a planned, healthy diet the majority of the time, Successful Losers can occasionally indulge in a craving – but they never go overboard.

Food addiction can really ruin your chances of becoming a Successful Loser. But if you cannot beat the enemy the best move is to join them. By carefully planning healthy menus Successful Losers include their favorite foods to help beat their cravings. So, what do they eat that you don't? What an intriguing question! Find out the answer in the next chapter

Chapter 8 in a nutshell

❖ Sugar is a simple carb, the consumption of which has increased dramatically over the last decades – contributing to the obesity epidemic and sugar addiction.

❖ Excessive consumption of sugar causes your brain to behave in ways similar to the brains of those who use drugs. Like any other addiction, the more you consume sugar, the more you body craves it.

❖ Among all these bad sugars, high-fructose corn syrup is the worst of them all – not only because it adds incredible amounts of empty calories to our diets, but also because it messes with the satiety signals going to your brain, causing you to stay hungry more often.

❖ Food addiction is a real threat to your attempt to become a Successful Loser. So, do what Successful Losers do and replace as much simple carbs as you can with smaller amounts of healthier treats (such as nuts and berries)!

[9]

What Successful Losers eat that you don't

Have you ever wondered why some people can eat a lot and not gain weight - while others are constantly struggling with their weight? I bet you have! There are many explanations for this phenomenon (as we have seen throughout this book), but they all have one thing in common: food choice. When choosing what to eat, Successful Losers follow a simple rule of thumb: Quantity, Times and Quality. Quantity stands for the portion size – remember that no food is entirely "good" or "bad" but any food in the wrong amount is potentially harmful. Times, as you can guess, stands for the number of meals you eat each day. Usually, it is recommended that you eat five to six times a day (breakfast,

snack, lunch, snack, dinner, and snack) at intervals of 3-4 hours –
Successful Losers really follow these rules! They eat more
frequently than the average Fat Joe – at least 5 times a day. Thus,
they are less likely to overeat at their next meal as they are not so
hungry, and chances are that they will choose healthier foods since
they know better than to use up their daily calorie intake in one
meal. Last but not least, Quality signifies the nutritional value and
caloric content of your food – not all healthy foods are low in
calories, but almost all foods low in calories are healthy.

*"When choosing what to eat, Successful Losers follow a
simple rule of thumb: Quantity, Times and Quality"*

Eating right is not rocket science! What makes it so confusing is
the number of misleading, erroneous or maliciously manipulated
information that we so often receive from the food industry and
media. The dieting industry insists on selling us a quick fix –
almost a miracle cure that we only need to buy and follow for a
short time to be slim forever. Nothing illustrates this better than
the popular fad diets. Fad diets are diets that promise you that you
will lose a large amount of weight in a short period of time, often
without changing your lifestyle habits. Fad diets are popular
because they seem easy and may work in the short term — but it
should be stressed that you usually regain the weight lost once you
stop dieting. Far too many people spend a lot of time and money
going from fad diet to fad diet without any long-term success.
Successful Losers – as we have learnt – never diet but instead
choose to permanently change their habits and their lifestyles – in
the process adopting a healthy diet that leads to weight loss and

better health over time. Their secrets are not super-advanced, but simply based on replacing unhealthy foods and behaviors with healthier ones. But unlike diets, these secrets work!

Scientists recently concluded a huge study of 2708 Successful Losers, examining how their eating and exercise behaviors had helped them to lose weight - and what had happened to these behaviors during the ten years following the initial weight loss [150]. Despite small changes in diet over time, what united these Successful Losers was their long-term maintenance of weight loss, a consistent continued low-calorie diet with a moderate fat intake, limited fast-food intake and high levels of physical activity. Only a minority consumed a low-carbohydrate diet – which again shows that it is the calorie content of the food that determines its obesogenic potential. In fact, most Successful Losers embraced carbohydrates as part of their health eating habits. Carbohydrates (with the exception of high-fructose corn syrup) are simply not the villains that popular diets want you to believe.

So, if not a miracle diet, what exactly do Successful Losers eat? Let's find out by looking in detail at a representative menu based on actual reported diets of Successful Losers – and compare to diets reported by patients who come to me because they struggle to lose weight.

Successful Loser's Menu	**Weight Regainer's Menu**
Breakfast – 310 kcal	Breakfast – 0 kcal
Oatmeal cinnamon swirl (1.5 oz)	Skips breakfast
Non-fat milk* (4 fl oz)	
Banana (1 medium)	
Coffee or tea (4 fl oz)	

Morning snack – 170 kcal
Cantaloupe melon (1 cup)
Blueberry cereal bars (1 serving)

Lunch – 550 kcal
Chicken ceasar wrap (1 serving)
Tangerine (1 medium)
Mineral water (3.5 fl oz)

Afternoon snack – 160 kcal
Non-fat yogurt (6 oz)
Red apple (1 small)

Dinner – 550 kcal
Whole-grain
pasta bolognese (10 oz)
Salad mix (1 1/2 cup)
Balsamic vinaigrette (1 tsp)
Mineral water (3.5 fl oz)

Night snack – 60 kcal
Apple (1 smal)

Total calories: 1800 kcal

Morning snack – 0 kcal
Skips snack

Lunch – 970 kcal
Macaroni and cheese (10 oz)
Soda (3.5 fl oz)

Afternoon snack – 290 kcal
M&Ms (1/2 cup)

Dinner** – 1000 kcal
Hamburger (5 oz)
French fries (4 oz)
Soda (3.5 fl oz)

Night snack – 0 kcal
Skip snack

Total calories: 2260 kcal

*For those who are lactose intolerant, choose lactose-free dairy products or soy-based products. ** Stops by at the drive-through of a junk food restaurant on the way home.

The two menus are clearly different! Indeed, they illustrate perfectly the difference between a healthy eating plan and an unhealthy one. But what is so special about the Successful Losers' plan? What is on their plate that is not on yours?

The answer to that question is simply that Successful Losers adopt healthy eating habits as part of their lifestyle. Indeed, all Successful

Losers know that the key to healthy eating is to make it as simple as possible. That's why they plan ahead, alternating between a limited number of recipes that are healthy, easy-to-make and delicious until they get used to their new diet. Most find it easier to eat healthily by having repetitive eating habits, at least for the first year or so. If you want to copy them, simply pick 15-20 easy-to-make, healthy recipes that you like, and choose one of these for every meal – you will soon learn to buy the right ingredients when at the supermarket. Make large portions and freeze leftovers as lunchboxes or for emergencies. Don't eat animal products every meal (try vegetarian food).

To manage, Successful Losers usually adopt a well-defined daily routine: they have the same breakfast at about the same time every day, they pack their planned lunch and take it wherever they go, and they have a regular workout schedule – as well as a spare set of athletic clothes in the trunk of their car. For example, on most days I eat breakfast around 7:30 am (half a cup of oatmeal with a glass of non-fat milk and half a banana sliced into my oatmeal, along with a cup of black coffee on the side). Sometimes on the weekend, I try to vary my breakfast menu by preparing an omelet or a whole-grain bagel with reduced fat cream cheese, again with a cup of coffee. For my daily lunch, I pack a whole-grain baguette sandwich (filled with grilled chicken breast, salad, mixed raw greens and 1 teaspoon olive oil) along with a small bag of mixed nuts and dry fruits, and a cup of non-fat yogurt – the latter I eat as a snack in the afternoon. For dinner, I have five favorite recipes that I consistently alternate. They are pumpkin soup, home-made tacos, grilled salmon with bulgur and vegetables, grilled chicken breast with bean salad, or vegetarian lasagna. None of which take more than 30 minutes to prepare, and all easily scalable so that I can cook for friends or for leftovers.

Successful Losers choose their food wisely

Good nutritional value is the result of countless chemical reactions in our bodies in response to the food we eat. To let the body use the formulas it knows best, choose foods that are rich in lean proteins, complex carbohydrates and healthy fats. With this in mind, Successful Losers choose to eat mostly natural foods that are unprocessed and unrefined. When you choose the right type of foods for your daily calories, you are not only going to lose weight but also make sure that your body has everything it needs to maintain the weight loss and preserve your health – to me, that sounds like a sweet deal. Remember, a calorie may be a calorie, but not all calories are delivered the same – as we have seen in Chapters 6 and 7.

Go back to basics: eat unprocessed whole foods!

Unprocessed or unrefined foods are foods that are eaten in their natural state – that is "whole". Calorie by calorie, these foods provide more dietary fiber, vitamins and minerals than do more processed varieties. For example, a fresh strawberry is an unprocessed food rich in vitamins, minerals and dietary fiber – but strawberry jam is processed and contains far fewer nutrients, being mostly made of sugar. Science has shown that whole grains (another unprocessed variety of common foodstuff) "play an important role in lowering the risk of chronic diseases, such as coronary heart disease, diabetes, and cancer, and also contribute to body weight management and gastrointestinal health" [151]. Those of us who consume more whole grain foods consistently weigh less than those who consume processed grain foods [152, 153]. Successful Losers never forget that dietary fibers, vitamins and minerals not only help reduce the risk of chronic diseases, but they are also key components of any healthy diet, essential for a well-functioning mind and body. Unprocessed foods may take some getting used to, but they are what our ancestors ate, what our bodies have been designed to ingest, and thus a powerful ally in the battle for weight loss and maintenance – just ask any Successful Loser!

On the other hand, heavily processed and refined foods such as potato chips, frozen meals, cookies, and white bread mostly contain trans fats and the type of carbohydrates that you want to avoid (remember the simple carbs?). Most, if not all, nutritional compounds (vitamins, minerals, dietary fiber and others) are lost during the refining process. So you end up consuming a product rich only in empty calories – precisely what you want to avoid! Not only do Successful Losers make unprocessed foods a central part of their eating habits, but they also avoid processed foods as much as possible.

Secret healthy foods

Who said that eating healthily has to be boring? As you know by now, a healthy diet is not composed of just vegetables and fruits – though they are a big part of it! A healthy diet consists of a variety of foods from each of the main nutrient groups (carbohydrates, proteins and fats), all eaten in moderation on a regular basis. There is a wide variety of healthy foods that are not so well-known – but that are delicious, easy to make and extremely healthy. Successful Losers know that by learning how to cook and season these super-foods they will have strong and tasty allies to help them reach their goals.

Following advice from Successful Losers, I have made a list of some of the world's super-foods to help you supercharge your diet, along with suggestions for how to serve them.

Avocado

This fruit native to Mexico has traveled the world and conquered an important place in the diet of Successful Losers – with good reason! Avocado consumers usually have a better overall diet – consuming more fruits and vegetables, dietary fiber, and healthy fats, while also eating less sugar. These healthy eating habits reflect on their figures as they have a lower body weight and a smaller waistline than do those of us who do not eat avocado regularly [154].

Nutritional value – avocado is packed with potassium, vitamin C, vitamin K, folate, dietary fiber and monounsaturated fats. However, too much of this good thing can add up to too many pounds of fat as avocado is relatively high in calories.

How to serve it – use it in salads, sandwiches, wraps, smoothies, or dips – also known in the Mexican cuisine as guacamole. Avocado is also a healthy replacement for butter spread (replace it with ripe avocado on your sandwich).

Beans and peas

Beans and peas come in many shapes, sizes and tastes – and are a staple food in most parts of the world (but unfortunately not in ours!) and one of the oldest cultivated plants. Because of this, it is estimated that there are over 40,000 types of beans – but only a few are readily available commercially. The most common are: green peas, yellow peas, chickpeas, pink beans, pinto beans, black beans, red beans, kidney beans and cranberry beans.

Nutritional value – beans and peas are a good source of iron, vitamin B6, folic acid, fiber, protein and unprocessed carbohydrates. Regular consumption of beans and peas has been linked to a lower body weight, as well as a smaller waistline.

How to serve it – beans and grains are a great match (try beans with brown rice, corn or tortillas) not only because they taste good together, but also because they complement each others' amino acid profiles. Other options used by Successful Losers are adding beans and/or peas to salads, soups, casseroles and even desserts!

Berries

With so many kinds and tastes, berries are nature's best sweet treats. They are also linked to a number of health benefits, such as improved heart health, decreased oxidative stress, and better blood lipids [155]. The most common berries in Western supermarkets are blueberries, strawberries, raspberries, cranberries and blackberries.

Nutritional value – low in calories and rich in antioxidants, phytochemicals, dietary fiber and vitamin C. Berries are best consumed fresh, but they also keep most of their nutritional value when frozen, or can be dried and eaten as healthy snacks.

How to serve it – add berries to your morning cereal, yogurt, smoothies, sauces, salads, or desserts – due to their sweetness, berries are a perfect choice for desserts.

Brown rice

Rice is the staple food for much of the world's population. Brown rice is unrefined, which means that it keeps the bran layer around the inner core grain, and along with it all of the natural nutrients stored there – unlike white rice, which is refined and in the process stripped of most of its nutrients. And more, brown rice may decrease diabetes risk, lower cholesterol and help maintain a healthy weight [156, 157].

Nutritional value – brown rice is an excellent source of selenium and manganese – a mineral that helps us digest fat and get the most from the proteins and carbohydrates that we eat.

How to serve it – brown rice is a versatile food that you can serve boiled or steamed. It goes well with beans, salads, woks and your choice of meat, chicken or fish.

Bulgur

Popular in the famously healthy Mediterranean cuisine, bulgur is made from wheat kernels and comes in fine, medium or coarse grades.

Nutritional value – bulgur is rich in dietary fibers and protein, as well as being cholesterol free.

How to serve it – after soaking bulgur in boiling water for 15 – 20 minutes (until tender), you can serve this delicious ingredient with salads, soups, and as a side dish for most meat and chicken. Use bulgur instead of potatoes – and serve it hot or cold!

Chicken breast

The chicken breast filet is probably one of the most popular cuts of meat – and with good reason. Using chickens raised in a humane way, slaughtered under hygienic conditions and not heavily processed (such as being soaked in salt water), it is not only really easy to prepare and season, but it is also relatively cheap compared to other types of meat (even when you take the above mentioned into consideration).

Nutritional value – chicken breast is high in protein, niacin, selenium, and vitamin B6 – but low in sodium and fat (when eaten skinless).

How to serve it – chicken breast is a versatile meat, and tastes great grilled, baked or steamed. It can also be incorporated into woks and casseroles. Personally, I really like grilled chicken breast marinated in garlic, lemon juice and oregano. One important tip: make sure that you remove the skin before you eat chicken – it is full of unsaturated fats that you want to avoid.

Eggs

Eggs probably are one of the most controversial foods in the world. This perfectly packaged and tasty ancient food was previously believed to cause a range of diseases from heart troubles to allergies. Luckily, current research has put eggs where they belong – on the list of must have super-foods that are not only healthy and an important part of a balanced diet, but that also can prevent and treat a number of health conditions. Regular egg consumption has now been linked to weight loss, increased satiety, reduced blood pressure, better fat and sugar control in diabetics and – when eaten in moderation – has no adverse effects on blood cholesterol levels [158, 159].

Nutritional value – eggs are a great source of protein, low in calories, as well as being rich in antioxidants, vitamin D, vitamin B12 and selenium.

How to serve it – eating an omelet for breakfast is a great way to start the day. Eggs can also be served boiled, scrambled, or incorporated into your cooking.

Leafy greens

I must confess that I like to feel full after a meal – and a great way that I have found to eat large portions without gaining weight is to add lots of leafy greens to my plate. I usually dedicate half of available plate space exclusively to leafy greens!

Nutritional value – leafy greens are a great source of dietary fiber, iron and calcium – and also contain vitamin C, vitamin K, folate and magnesium. They have virtually no fat or calories – so don't eat them exclusively.

How to serve it – super low in calories, these leaves add tons of flavor and texture to salads, soups, casseroles, and woks – or as a side dish to almost any food.

Low-fat dairy products

Dairy products are key ingredients in most Western cuisines. In fact, they are used so often that for some people – including myself – it is hard to imagine life without them! The good news is that you do not have to! By choosing low-fat or fat-free dairy products, you can enjoy the benefits without the harmful bad fats and extra calories. For those of us who are intolerant to lactose, there are now a great variety of dairy products free from both fat and lactose – but if you are allergic to milk protein you know by now to skip dairy products altogether.

Nutritional value – dairy products are undoubtedly the best source of calcium in the diet, and are also a good source of protein and vitamin D. When consuming low-fat or fat-free dairy products, the amount of saturated fat is almost zero.

How to serve it – depending on the type of dairy product you are consuming, you will generally drink it (milk or yogurt), have it with bread (cheese or butter) or simply mix it with your food while cooking.

Nuts and seeds

Eating nuts and seeds regularly is a great way to pack vitamins and minerals into your diet. And more, regular consumption of nuts and seeds has been linked to a decreased risk of heart disease and a lower body weight [160] [161].

Nutritional value – nuts and seeds are a great source of protein, vitamin E, vitamin B6, folic acid and niacin, as well as dietary fiber, and antioxidants such as omega-3. But don't overeat – these foods are highly caloric, especially if mixed with sugar (it is best to avoid the confectionary or salted types of nuts). Usually, one handful (1 oz) a day is enough to get all the nutritional benefits without compromising your waistline.

How to serve it – nuts and seeds are great snack food, not only because of their outstanding nutritional value, but also because they are so practical to carry around. They can also be added to salad, casseroles, and woks.

Pumpkin

Native to North America, this exquisite fruit is, unfortunately, to many people a mere decoration used at Halloween and forgotten during the rest of the year. However, pumpkin is a nutritional powerhouse, with scientific studies showing that it prevents fatigue and lowers blood sugar, at least in animals [162, 163].

Nutritional value – pumpkins of most kinds are an excellent source of vitamin A, vitamin C, riboflavin, potassium, copper, manganese and dietary fiber. This sweet treat is also very low in calories and fats. Enjoy it!

How to serve it – pumpkin can be served as soup, pie or puree, as well as baked, boiled or steamed and makes a great addition to casseroles, woks, and salads.

Quinoa

Quinoa is a grass-like crop cultivated in the Andes for thousands of years. Recently, this humble food has attracted a lot of attention due to its powerful nutritional content and blend.

Nutritional value – quinoa is one of the only plant foods that offer a complete selection of protein (i.e. all of the essential amino acids that our body cannot produce on its own). Quinoa is a great source of complex carbohydrates, and the best whole grain source of potassium. Also, quinoa can assist weight loss and maintenance by keeping you fuller longer – due to its high content of dietary fiber.

How to serve it – the quinoa seeds should be boiled in water for about 10-15 minutes. You know that they are ready when the germ separates from the seed! Successful Losers use quinoa to replace white rice and other refined grains. It can also be incorporated cold into soups, salads, and baked goods.

Seafood

Seafood is any edible thing coming from the sea, but undoubtedly the most common one is fish in all its variety. However, fish is far from being the only delicious and nutritious seafood! Other popular types of seafood are shrimp, clams, and oysters.

Nutritional value – seafood is a great ally when working to lose weight, as it is generally low in calories and rich in a number of nutrients. Most seafood is rich in omega-3 fatty acids (which are a friendly type of fat), lean protein, and also a good source of selenium, vitamin D, vitamin B12, zinc, and iodine. Be aware that some seafood (including shrimp and crawfish) are very low in calories – but rich in cholesterol, so if you need to watch your cholesterol do not eat these more than once a week.

How to serve it – seafood can be a key ingredient served in many dishes: from salads, soups, and casseroles to woks. Serve it fried, grilled or raw with pasta, bulgur, brown rice or quinoa. Many people do not like seafood – but with so many to choose from, and so many ways to cook it, I bet that you can find one that you will love!

Sweet potatoes

Can't live without potatoes? Well, you don't have to! Sweet potatoes are a great replacement for regular potatoes. Not only do they taste better, they also provide a whole spectrum of nutrients that regular potatoes lack.

Nutritional value – sweet potatoes are not only super low in saturated fat and cholesterol, but they are also a good source of dietary fiber, vitamin A, vitamin C, vitamin B6, potassium, and manganese.

How to serve it – sweet potatoes can substitute for regular potatoes in most recipes, or can be served baked, boiled, roasted, pureed or in a casserole.

Water

Almost 2/3 of our bodies are water. So it's not surprising that we daily need adequate amounts of water to live. In our bodies, water carries vital nutrients to cells, gets rid of toxins, regulates our body temperature, hydrates the skin and tissues, and prevents constipation – just to name a few of the many essential functions of water.

Nutritional value – despite not containing any calories, and very few nutrients, water is central to maintaining good health. But what exactly is the daily adequate amount of water? The answer depends on your sex, age, level of physical activity, environment (you need more fluids if you live in a place with hot weather) and much else besides. Fortunately, you come equipped with thirst – the body's own sensitive regulator of hydration. If you really want a number, in general 8-10 glasses of water daily covers most people's needs.

How to serve it – drink water with your meals instead of juice or soda – and remember to also drink it between meals and at snack times. If you think plain water is too boring, try adding a few drops of fruit.

Spice things up! Add taste, not calories

Who said that making foods taste great has to be about calorie rich cream, butter, and sugar? For thousands of years, our ancestors and every known civilization has collected and grown herbs and spices to add flavors and a myriad of health benefits to their food – all without any additional calories. In fact, Successful Losers know that natural seasonings actually decrease the amount of calories you eat if they are used to replace excess sugar, salt or fat. Below is a list of my personal favorite seasonings.

Garlic

Not everyone likes it, but garlic is one of my all time favorites! Not only for its exquisite taste, but also for its content of powerful disease-fighting substances that can battle cancer cells, prevent high blood sugar, lower cholesterol, and act as potent anti-inflammatory agents [164]. On top of that, regular consumption of garlic can also lower blood pressure.

How to serve it – just add fresh crushed or chopped garlic to anything from sauces and soups to casseroles, pastas, fish, meat, and poultry dishes.

Chili pepper

Red and hot – who can resist that? When consumed regularly, a group of substances in chili pepper called capsaicinoids have been demonstrated to increased energy expenditure, reduce abdominal fat, and decreased hunger and calorie consumption [165] – with such a strong taste no one will be able to wolf down double portions or overeat! That's what I call a weight loss ally!

How to serve it – if you are not used to eating spicy food, I suggest starting slow by adding chili little by little until you find the right amount for you. Try it in soups, sauces, casserole, stews, marinades, and of course with salsa or beans.

Oregano

Oregano is an important part of the Italian cuisine – it is what makes pizza taste like pizza. It can be used fresh or dried to add an aromatic flavor to food.
How to serve it – add it in egg dishes, pastas, pizzas, tomato sauce and sandwiches. A great substitute for salt!

Ginger

This slightly hot spice originally comes from southern China – but has by now made its way to all corners of the world. Despite its great taste ginger has many health benefits, such as decreasing bad cholesterol. In addition, consuming ginger during four weeks is enough to reduce body weight and increase the good cholesterol – at least in rat studies [166].

How to serve it – add it freshly grated to casseroles, stews, soups, sauces, baked goods – or even make ginger tea.

Cinnamon

Like most people, I love the smell and taste of cinnamon in the morning! I have it every day mixed into my oatmeal at breakfast. It tastes so good that I don't even add sugar anymore. It not only tastes great, but it has also been proven to have therapeutic effects by lowering sugar, fat and cholesterol in the blood [167] [168].

How to serve it – add it instead of sugar to hot beverages such as coffee, hot chocolate or tea, or into porridge, baked goods, cereal or casseroles.

Food allergies and intolerance

For those of you who have a food allergy, or are intolerant of certain foods – such as gluten or lactose – these items must be removed from your diet regardless of how much you like them or how healthy they have been shown to be. To you, they will inevitably do you more harm than good. Luckily, most foods today are available in special formats for those who cannot eat the regular variety. For example, those with lactose intolerance can now choose dairy products that are low in lactose, while those allergic to gluten can buy gluten free bread.

[10]

To err is human, but to persist to err is just stupid!

How wonderful life would be if we could always perform at our best, never make any mistakes and always get it right on the very first try! We would never get hurt, disappointed or embarrassed! But from an early age, we learn that life does not work in this way. And sometimes, despite your best efforts, everything that could go wrong indeed goes wrong! What to do then? Give up your hopes and dreams? Settle for less than you can be? Or learn from experience and start fresh with your newfound knowledge about yourself? I bet you can guess which one Successful Losers go for!

From time to time, we all make mistakes! Beating yourself up about them will only undermine your self-confidence (and as we have seen, that will only take you further from your goals). What to do then? As Al Franken wrote "Mistakes are a part of being human. Appreciate your mistakes for what they are: precious life lessons that can only be learned the hard way!" Sure, you did everything right except for that one little mistake – maybe overeating at your nephew's birthday party and then feeling bad about your "weakness", or skipping your gym classes three weeks in a row and ending up feeling like a failure, or suddenly gaining all the weight that you had lost over a long and arduous weight-loss program. I know the bitter taste of feeling like a failure is not a good one – believe me I've been there! But as all Successful Losers know, the road to success is not a smooth ride; it is made up of innumerable challenges and setbacks – all of which have to be faced. What distinguishes Successful Losers from all others is not that they never fail – but how they manage to face the obstacles and deal constructively with the inevitable setbacks. Successful Losers know how to deal constructively with their unavoidable setbacks, learn from them, and get back on track in no time! And so can you!

The all or nothing trap

To many people, weight loss and a healthy lifestyle are all-or-nothing commitments – either you do everything right, or you do nothing at all. Big mistake! In my experience, this is in fact one of the main reasons for why so many people fail when trying to lose weight! Aiming for perfection sets you up to fail. To not make a single mistake in life is simply not possible – or human for that matter! If you subscribe to the all or nothing philosophy, when faced with anything less than a 100% success rate you may fall into guilty despair convinced that you are a failure, which increases the chance of making another mistake that can in fact easily take you right back to your old and unhealthy habits. The sooner you accept that you are going to slip up every now and then, the better prepared you are going to be to deal with setbacks when they occur. Instead of aiming for perfection, you should be focusing on continuous improvement – and instead of despairing at your mistakes and seeking to place blame, you should be concentrating on damage control and on quickly bouncing back without taking damage to your health or self-esteem.

"Aiming for perfection sets you up to fail"

Since you are now developing a new, healthy lifestyle built to last – not following someone else's diet rulebook – you can do things differently. Healthy living is a lifelong process of continuous effort and evolution – which is why it clearly requires a lot of trial and error. Working as a dietitian, I have yet to meet a single person that has had an easy, straight and one-way journey when achieving lasting weight loss. Rather, the usual process is two steps forwards, one step back. But, with each step back, if you are willing to learn you can get invaluable information about who you are and how you work – knowledge that you then apply to take two more steps towards your goals.

Get to know yourself!

As we have seen in Secret V, knowledge is power! The more you know and understand something, the better equipped you are to deal with it. This goes doubly when applied to you! Have you ever wondered why you keep making the same mistakes over and over again? Could it be that you need to learn to say "no, thanks" when offered food, become more attuned to how your emotions drive you to use food as a way of comforting yourself, or learn to differentiate between your body signaling a genuine need for rest and just signaling a wish to avoid working out due to laziness? The more you know about how your body and brain works, what you prefer, when you feel more (or less) energetic, and what triggers your overeating – along with all the other issues that get in the way of reaching your goals – the better you will understand why you are where you are, and what to do about it!

Susan R., a 34 years old full-time mother of four young children told me that her main challenge was to stop eating her children's leftovers. "I come from a family where wasting food is almost a sin, so I used to feel like I had the moral obligation to eat whatever my kids left on their plates. And I did!" As a result, Susan R. watched the pounds pile on faster and faster after each pregnancy. "When I finally realized what I was doing to my body, I knew that I had to stop that terrible habit of mine. After much trial and error, I started to only put the amount of food that I know the children will eat on their plates. Not only did this prevent me from feeling bad about wasting food, but it also enabled me to lose more than 25 pounds. It's a win-win situation!"

If you keep making the same mistake over and over again, chances are that you are sabotaging yourself. If that is the case, I strongly suggest that you – yourself or with help – find out both why you subconsciously believe this is to your advantage, and in which subtle (or not so subtle) ways you are ruining your chances to attain the body you have always wanted.

This is a complex issue about which a whole other book may be written. However, to get you started, I have listed some questions below that may help you to understand yourself better and discover strategies to cope with your uncertainty. As always, the key to avoiding self-sabotage in the future is to understand why it happens (and there is a why) through getting to know yourself better.

Overeating

* When in time am I more prone to overeating? In what setting?
* When I overeat, in which physical and emotional state am I?
* What could/should I do instead of overeating?
* What do I gain by indulging in my short-term wishes? Is the gain more desirable than achieving my long-term goals?
* What are the long-term effects of my overeating on my health, relationships and activities that I find pleasure in?

Emotional eating

* When I eat for comfort, in which emotional state am I?
* What feeling do I wish to get when I eat for comfort?
* What situations and feelings are most likely to trigger a need to eat for comfort? Hunger/loneliness/boredom/ stress/sadness/happiness/etc.
* What do I get by indulging in my short-term wish for comfort? Is it going to take me closer from or further my goals?

❖ What could/should I do instead of emotional eating?

Avoiding physical activity

❖ When in time and in what setting am I more prone to procrastinate and be sedentary?

❖ Do I really not have time for regular, planned physical activity - or do I not want to make time for it? Why?

❖ How would physical activity on a regular basis affect my feelings of tiredness/stress/boredom/sadness/depression?

❖ Am I genuinely in need of physical rest, or am I procrastinating/tired/lazy?

❖ What do I get by indulging in my short-term wish to avoid exertion? Is avoiding regular physical activity in the short -term going to take me closer to or further from my long-term goals?

We are all different and unique individuals with different personalities, priorities, attitudes, and circumstances. There is no one solution that fits everyone, but by honestly answering these questions to yourself, you will shed some light on the unconscious actions and preferences that may be preventing you from achieving your goals and becoming a Successful Loser.

Give yourself a break

So, you screwed up again! After spending all that time setting attainable goals, working on your eating habits and physical activity, getting to know yourself better and figuring out the reasons behind your self-sabotage. However good your intentions and careful your planning, chances are that you will still slip back into your old habits every now and then! How frustrating, huh? Not to mention the impact it can have on your self-esteem! But it does not have to be a catastrophe if you focus on finding empowering ways to deal with the situation and learn from it.

There will always be challenges and failures on the path to achieving your goals – and I can guarantee that at some point you are going to make some very bad decisions and do everything that you now know you are supposed to avoid! But these events are not as important as what you are going to do after they happen. Are you going to let them throw you completely off track and reduce you to a state of despair? We all make mistakes and the trick when that happens is to ask yourself how you can prevent that particular bad thing from happening again. You need to be compassionate with yourself, forgiving the occasional slip while trying very hard to not let it happen again. The act of forgiving oneself has been much studied, and exercising this option not only provides you with better overall physical health, but also with better mental health [169, 170]. And more, when you do not forgive yourself, you instead tend to get angry, which in turn leads to stress that contributes to making you fat [171].

Next time you realize that you have screwed up, focus on identifying why so that you won't make the same mistake again. Instead of berating yourself and dwelling on the past, focus all your energy on returning to your original plan. Remember that if you are not failing once in a while, you are not trying hard enough!

This time can really be different!

After many attempts to lose weight, you may ask "what is the point of even trying?" or "even if I succeed at first I will end up slipping back again!" Sounds familiar? If so, now is the time to change your internal dialogue to a more empowering one. If you are like most people, you have probably tried to lose weight many times. Indeed, nearly 91% of Successful Losers reported that they tried unsuccessfully to lose weight before they managed to achieve a healthy weight and stay slim [7]. Preventing small regains from turning into larger relapses is critical to success amongst Successful Losers.

So, remember that it's not unusual to occasionally lose track of your weight-loss program and slip back into old patterns of unhealthy eating and minimal exercise. In fact, given how complicated life can be, you should expect mistakes to happen and have a plan in place to rapidly get back on track when slip-ups occur. It takes time and regular practice for your new healthy behaviors to become habits. Above all, realize that you're not a failure. Reverting to old behaviors doesn't mean that all hope is lost. It just means that you need to improve your plan, recharge your motivation, recommit to your program and return to healthy behaviors [172] – that's what Successful Losers do!

I hope that you have enjoyed reading this book as much as I have enjoyed writing it! Remember that only reading this (or any other) book will not turn you into a Successful Loser overnight. It is now up to you to put your new knowledge into practice! As we have learnt, there are no short-cuts, magic pills or miracle diets – but I am convinced that this is exactly why the methods outlined here actually work so well! The ability to transform your life is literally in your hands, and your decision to master your environment and lead a healthy lifestyle will make all the difference. If you think like a Successful Loser and act like a Successful Loser you will become one too!

Chapter 10 in a nutshell

❖ Making mistakes is part of the journey to becoming a Successful Loser. But to keep on making the same mistake is just stupid. Learn from your mistakes and move on!

❖ Aiming for perfection is a sure way to fail. Instead, aim for constant improvement!

❖ If you keep making the same mistake over and over again, chances are that you are sabotaging yourself. What are you afraid you will lose by changing?

❖ All Successful Losers have failed – and still do – a number of times, but when it happens they do not fall victim to self-pity but instead decide to focus on how to get back on track.

About the author

Before becoming a certified dietitian with a PhD in clinical nutrition, Thiane Axelsson was an uncontrolled eater in a permanent fight with the scales. She lost and gained weight time and time again until she finally hit upon the secrets of permanent healthy weight loss. Out of simple self-preservation, she has always been fascinated by why we eat what we eat, and how food affects our lives. Helping people to lose weight in a healthy and sustainable way has become a passion, and the author's life project.

References

1. Wing, R. R., and Phelan, S. (2005) Long-term weight loss maintenance, *Am J Clin Nutr 82*, 222S-225S.
2. Polivy, J. (1996) Psychological consequences of food restriction., *J Am Diet Assoc 96*, 589-592; quiz 593-584.
3. Pederson Mussell, M., Mitchell, J. E., Fenna, C. J., Crosby, R. D., Miller, J. P., and Hoberman, H. M. (1997) A comparison of onset of binge eating versus dieting in the development of bulimia nervosa., *Int J Eat Disord 21*, 353-360.
4. Elfhag, K., and Rössner, S. (2005) Who succeeds in maintaining weight loss? A conceptual review of factors associated with weight loss maintenance and weight regain., *Obes Rev 6*, 67-85.
5. Chambers, J. A., and Swanson, V. (2011) Stories of weight management: Factors associated with successful and unsuccessful weight maintenance., *Br J Health Psychol*.
6. McGuire, M. T., Wing, R. R., Klem, M. L., and Hill, J. O. (1999) Behavioral strategies of individuals who have maintained long-term weight losses., *Obes Res 7*, 334-341.
7. Klem, M. L., Wing, R. R., McGuire, M. T., Seagle, H. M., and Hill, J. O. (1997) A descriptive study of individuals

successful at long-term maintenance of substantial weight loss., *Am J Clin Nutr 66*, 239-246.

8.		Choquet, H., and Meyre, D. (2011) Genetics of Obesity: What have we Learned?, *Curr Genomics 12*, 169-179.

9.		Speliotes, E. K., Willer, C. J., Berndt, S. I., Monda, K. L., Thorleifsson, G., Jackson, A. U., Allen, H. L., Lindgren, C. M., Luan, J., Mägi, R., Randall, J. C., Vedantam, S., Winkler, T. W., Qi, L., Workalemahu, T., Heid, I. M., Steinthorsdottir, V., Stringham, H. M., Weedon, M. N., Wheeler, E., Wood, A. R., Ferreira, T., Weyant, R. J., Segrè, A. V., Estrada, K., Liang, L., Nemesh, J., Park, J. H., Gustafsson, S., Kilpeläinen, T. O., Yang, J., Bouatia-Naji, N., Esko, T., Feitosa, M. F., Kutalik, Z., Mangino, M., Raychaudhuri, S., Scherag, A., Smith, A. V., Welch, R., Zhao, J. H., Aben, K. K., Absher, D. M., Amin, N., Dixon, A. L., Fisher, E., Glazer, N. L., Goddard, M. E., Heard-Costa, N. L., Hoesel, V., Hottenga, J. J., Johansson, A., Johnson, T., Ketkar, S., Lamina, C., Li, S., Moffatt, M. F., Myers, R. H., Narisu, N., Perry, J. R., Peters, M. J., Preuss, M., Ripatti, S., Rivadeneira, F., Sandholt, C., Scott, L. J., Timpson, N. J., Tyrer, J. P., van Wingerden, S., Watanabe, R. M., White, C. C., Wiklund, F., Barlassina, C., Chasman, D. I., Cooper, M. N., Jansson, J. O., Lawrence, R. W., Pellikka, N., Prokopenko, I., Shi, J., Thiering, E., Alavere, H., Alibrandi, M. T., Almgren, P., Arnold, A. M., Aspelund, T., Atwood, L. D., Balkau, B., Balmforth, A. J., Bennett, A. J., Ben-Shlomo, Y., Bergman, R. N., Bergmann, S., Biebermann, H., Blakemore, A. I., Boes, T., Bonnycastle, L. L., Bornstein, S. R., Brown, M. J., Buchanan, T. A., Busonero, F., Campbell, H., Cappuccio, F. P., Cavalcanti-Proença, C., Chen, Y. D., Chen, C. M., Chines, P. S., Clarke, R., Coin, L., Connell, J., Day, I. N., den Heijer, M., Duan, J., Ebrahim, S., Elliott, P., Elosua, R., Eiriksdottir, G., Erdos, M. R., Eriksson, J. G., Facheris, M. F., Felix, S. B., Fischer-Posovszky, P., Folsom, A. R., Friedrich, N., Freimer, N. B., Fu, M., Gaget, S., Gejman, P. V., Geus, E. J., Gieger, C., Gjesing, A. P., Goel, A., Goyette, P., Grallert, H., Grässler, J., Greenawalt, D. M., Groves, C. J., Gudnason, V., Guiducci, C.,

Hartikainen, A. L., Hassanali, N., Hall, A. S., Havulinna, A. S., Hayward, C., Heath, A. C., Hengstenberg, C., Hicks, A. A., Hinney, A., Hofman, A., Homuth, G., Hui, J., Igl, W., Iribarren, C., Isomaa, B., Jacobs, K. B., Jarick, I., Jewell, E., John, U., Jørgensen, T., Jousilahti, P., Jula, A., Kaakinen, M., Kajantie, E., Kaplan, L. M., Kathiresan, S., Kettunen, J., Kinnunen, L., Knowles, J. W., Kolcic, I., König, I. R., Koskinen, S., Kovacs, P., Kuusisto, J., Kraft, P., Kvaløy, K., Laitinen, J., Lantieri, O., Lanzani, C., Launer, L. J., Lecoeur, C., Lehtimäki, T., Lettre, G., Liu, J., Lokki, M. L., Lorentzon, M., Luben, R. N., Ludwig, B., Manunta, P., Marek, D., Marre, M., Martin, N. G., McArdle, W. L., McCarthy, A., McKnight, B., Meitinger, T., Melander, O., Meyre, D., Midthjell, K., Montgomery, G. W., Morken, M. A., Morris, A. P., Mulic, R., Ngwa, J. S., Nelis, M., Neville, M. J., Nyholt, D. R., O'Donnell, C. J., O'Rahilly, S., Ong, K. K., Oostra, B., Paré, G., Parker, A. N., Perola, M., Pichler, I., Pietiläinen, K. H., Platou, C. G., Polasek, O., Pouta, A., Rafelt, S., Raitakari, O., Rayner, N. W., Ridderstråle, M., Rief, W., Ruokonen, A., Robertson, N. R., Rzehak, P., Salomaa, V., Sanders, A. R., Sandhu, M. S., Sanna, S., Saramies, J., Savolainen, M. J., Scherag, S., Schipf, S., Schreiber, S., Schunkert, H., Silander, K., Sinisalo, J., Siscovick, D. S., Smit, J. H., Soranzo, N., Sovio, U., Stephens, J., Surakka, I., Swift, A. J., Tammesoo, M. L., Tardif, J. C., Teder-Laving, M., Teslovich, T. M., Thompson, J. R., Thomson, B., Tönjes, A., Tuomi, T., van Meurs, J. B., van Ommen, G. J., Vatin, V., Viikari, J., Visvikis-Siest, S., Vitart, V., Vogel, C. I., Voight, B. F., Waite, L. L., Wallaschofski, H., Walters, G. B., Widen, E., Wiegand, S., Wild, S. H., Willemsen, G., Witte, D. R., Witteman, J. C., Xu, J., Zhang, Q., Zgaga, L., Ziegler, A., Zitting, P., Beilby, J. P., Farooqi, I. S., Hebebrand, J., Huikuri, H. V., James, A. L., Kähönen, M., Levinson, D. F., Macciardi, F., Nieminen, M. S., Ohlsson, C., Palmer, L. J., Ridker, P. M., Stumvoll, M., Beckmann, J. S., Boeing, H., Boerwinkle, E., Boomsma, D. I., Caulfield, M. J., Chanock, S. J., Collins, F. S., Cupples, L. A., Smith, G. D., Erdmann, J., Froguel, P., Grönberg, H., Gyllensten, U., Hall,

P., Hansen, T., Harris, T. B., Hattersley, A. T., Hayes, R. B., Heinrich, J., Hu, F. B., Hveem, K., Illig, T., Jarvelin, M. R., Kaprio, J., Karpe, F., Khaw, K. T., Kiemeney, L. A., Krude, H., Laakso, M., Lawlor, D. A., Metspalu, A., Munroe, P. B., Ouwehand, W. H., Pedersen, O., Penninx, B. W., Peters, A., Pramstaller, P. P., Quertermous, T., Reinehr, T., Rissanen, A., Rudan, I., Samani, N. J., Schwarz, P. E., Shuldiner, A. R., Spector, T. D., Tuomilehto, J., Uda, M., Uitterlinden, A., Valle, T. T., Wabitsch, M., Waeber, G., Wareham, N. J., Watkins, H., Wilson, J. F., Wright, A. F., Zillikens, M. C., Chatterjee, N., McCarroll, S. A., Purcell, S., Schadt, E. E., Visscher, P. M., Assimes, T. L., Borecki, I. B., Deloukas, P., Fox, C. S., Groop, L. C., Haritunians, T., Hunter, D. J., Kaplan, R. C., Mohlke, K. L., O'Connell, J. R., Peltonen, L., Schlessinger, D., Strachan, D. P., van Duijn, C. M., Wichmann, H. E., Frayling, T. M., Thorsteinsdottir, U., Abecasis, G. R., Barroso, I., Boehnke, M., Stefansson, K., North, K. E., McCarthy, M. I., Hirschhorn, J. N., Ingelsson, E., Loos, R. J., MAGIC, and Consortium, P. (2010) Association analyses of 249,796 individuals reveal 18 new loci associated with body mass index., *Nat Genet 42*, 937-948.

10.   Hu, F. B. (2011) Globalization of diabetes: the role of diet, lifestyle, and genes., *Diabetes Care 34*, 1249-1257.

11.   Hu, F. B., Li, T. Y., Colditz, G. A., Willett, W. C., and Manson, J. E. (2003) Television watching and other sedentary behaviors in relation to risk of obesity and type 2 diabetes mellitus in women., *JAMA 289*, 1785-1791.

12.   Hu, F. B. (2003) Sedentary lifestyle and risk of obesity and type 2 diabetes., *Lipids 38*, 103-108.

13.   Avena, N. M., Rada, P., and Hoebel, B. G. (2008) Evidence for sugar addiction: behavioral and neurochemical effects of intermittent, excessive sugar intake., *Neurosci Biobehav Rev 32*, 20-39.

14.   Erlanson-Albertsson, C. (2005) Appetite regulation and energy balance., *Acta Paediatr Suppl 94*, 40-41.

15.	Maller, O., and Desor, J. A. (1973) Effect of taste on ingestion by human newborns., *Symp Oral Sens Percept*, 279-291.

16.	Beauchamp, G. K., and Mennella, J. A. (2011) Flavor perception in human infants: development and functional significance., *Digestion 83 Suppl 1*, 1-6.

17.	Wansink, B., Bascoul, G., and Chen, G. T. (2006) The sweet tooth hypothesis: how fruit consumption relates to snack consumption., *Appetite 47*, 107-110.

18.	Canetti, L., Bachar, E., and Berry, E. M. (2002) Food and emotion., *Behav Processes 60*, 157-164.

19.	Troisi, J. D., and Gabriel, S. (2011) Chicken soup really is good for the soul: "comfort food" fulfills the need to belong., *Psychol Sci 22*, 747-753.

20.	Zeeck, A., Stelzer, N., Linster, H. W., Joos, A., and Hartmann, A. (2010) Emotion and eating in binge eating disorder and obesity., *Eur Eat Disord Rev.*

21.	French, S. A. (2003) Pricing effects on food choices., *J Nutr 133*, 841S-843S.

22.	French, S. A., Jeffery, R. W., Story, M., Breitlow, K. K., Baxter, J. S., Hannan, P., and Snyder, M. P. (2001) Pricing and promotion effects on low-fat vending snack purchases: the CHIPS Study., *Am J Public Health 91*, 112-117.

23.	Birch, L. L., and Marlin, D. W. (1982) I don't like it; I never tried it: effects of exposure on two-year-old children's food preferences., *Appetite 3*, 353-360.

24.	Christakis, N. A., and Fowler, J. H. (2007) The spread of obesity in a large social network over 32 years., *N Engl J Med 357*, 370-379.

25.	Flegal, K. M., Carroll, M. D., Kuczmarski, R. J., and Johnson, C. L. (1998) Overweight and obesity in the United States: prevalence and trends, 1960-1994., *Int J Obes Relat Metab Disord 22*, 39-47.

26.	Centers for Disease Control and Prevention, C. Overweight and Obesity. US Obesity Trends. Trends by State 1985–

2010.http://www.cdc.gov/obesity/data/trends.html.
Accessed on 12th December 2011.

27.	Preventing Chronic Diseases: a Vital Investment: Geneva, W. H. O., 2005.

28.	Wang, Y., Beydoun, M. A., Liang, L., Caballero, B., and Kumanyika, S. K. (2008) Will all Americans become overweight or obese? estimating the progression and cost of the US obesity epidemic., *Obesity (Silver Spring) 16*, 2323-2330.

29.	(CDC), C. f. D. C. a. P. (2011) Vital signs: prevalence, treatment, and control of high levels of low-density lipoprotein cholesterol--United States, 1999-2002 and 2005-200., *MMWR Morb Mortal Wkly Rep 60*, 109-114.

30.	Garber, A. J. (2011) Obesity and type 2 diabetes: which patients are at risk?, *Diabetes Obes Metab.*

31.	Gaesser, G. A., Angadi, S. S., and Sawyer, B. J. (2011) Exercise and diet, independent of weight loss, improve cardiometabolic risk profile in overweight and obese individuals., *Phys Sportsmed 39*, 87-97.

32.	Garfinkel, L. (1985) Overweight and cancer., *Ann Intern Med 103*, 1034-1036.

33.	Jia, H., and Lubetkin, E. I. (2010) Obesity-related quality-adjusted life years lost in the U.S. from 1993 to 2008., *Am J Prev Med 39*, 220-227.

34.	Lake, A., and Townshend, T. (2006) Obesogenic environments: exploring the built and food environments., *J R Soc Promot Health 126*, 262-267.

35.	Schwartz, J., and Byrd-Bredbenner, C. (2006) Portion distortion: typical portion sizes selected by young adults., *J Am Diet Assoc 106*, 1412-1418.

36.	Lowe, M. R. (2003) Self-regulation of energy intake in the prevention and treatment of obesity: is it feasible?, *Obes Res 11 Suppl*, 44S-59S.

37.	Farias, M. M., Cuevas, A. M., and Rodriguez, F. (2011) Set-point theory and obesity., *Metab Syndr Relat Disord 9*, 85-89.

38.   Bouchard, C., Tremblay, A., Després, J. P., Nadeau, A., Lupien, P. J., Thériault, G., Dussault, J., Moorjani, S., Pinault, S., and Fournier, G. (1990) The response to long-term overfeeding in identical twins., *N Engl J Med 322*, 1477-1482.

39.   Bouchard, C., Tremblay, A., Després, J. P., Nadeau, A., Lupien, P. J., Moorjani, S., Thériault, G., and Kim, S. Y. (1996) Overfeeding in identical twins: 5-year postoverfeeding results., *Metabolism 45*, 1042-1050.

40.   Robinson, T. N. (1999) Reducing children's television viewing to prevent obesity: a randomized controlled trial., *JAMA 282*, 1561-1567.

41.   Lean, M. E., Han, T. S., and Morrison, C. E. (1995) Waist circumference as a measure for indicating need for weight management, *BMJ 311*, 158-161.

42.   Prochaska, J. O., DiClemente, C. C., and Norcross, J. C. (1992) In search of how people change. Applications to addictive behaviors, *Am Psychol 47*, 1102-1114.

43.   Shilts, M. K., Horowitz, M., and Townsend, M. S. (2004) Goal setting as a strategy for dietary and physical activity behavior change: a review of the literature., *Am J Health Promot 19*, 81-93.

44.   DeWalt, D. A., Davis, T. C., Wallace, A. S., Seligman, H. K., Bryant-Shilliday, B., Arnold, C. L., Freburger, J., and Schillinger, D. (2009) Goal setting in diabetes self-management: taking the baby steps to success., *Patient Educ Couns 77*, 218-223.

45.   Brown, V. A., Bartholomew, L. K., and Naik, A. D. (2007) Management of chronic hypertension in older men: an exploration of patient goal-setting., *Patient Educ Couns 69*, 93-99.

46.   Foster, G. D., Makris, A. P., and Bailer, B. A. (2005) Behavioral treatment of obesity., *Am J Clin Nutr 82*, 230S-235S.

47.   Bodenheimer, T., and Handley, M. A. (2009) Goal-setting for behavior change in primary care: an

exploration and status report., *Patient Educ Couns 76*, 174-180.

48.   Campfield, L. A., Smith, F. J., and Burn, P. (1998) Strategies and potential molecular targets for obesity treatment., *Science 280*, 1383-1387.

49.   Goldstein, D. J. (1992) Beneficial health effects of modest weight loss., *Int J Obes Relat Metab Disord 16*, 397-415.

50.   Pearson, E. S. (2011) Goal setting as a health behavior change strategy in overweight and obese adults: A systematic literature review examining intervention components., *Patient Educ Couns.*

51.   Estabrooks, P. A., Nelson, C. C., Xu, S., King, D., Bayliss, E. A., Gaglio, B., Nutting, P. A., and Glasgow, R. E. (2005) The frequency and behavioral outcomes of goal choices in the self-management of diabetes., *Diabetes Educ 31*, 391-400.

52.   Ryan, R. M., and Deci, E. L. (2000) Self-determination theory and the facilitation of intrinsic motivation, social development, and well-being., *Am Psychol 55*, 68-78.

53.   Locke, E. A., and Latham, G. P. (2002) Building a practically useful theory of goal setting and task motivation. A 35-year odyssey., *Am Psychol 57*, 705-717.

54.   Dennis, K. E., and Goldberg, A. P. (1996) Weight control self-efficacy types and transitions affect weight-loss outcomes in obese women., *Addict Behav 21*, 103-116.

55.   Nir, Z., and Neumann, L. (1995) Relationship among self-esteem, internal-external locus of control, and weight change after participation in a weight reduction program., *J Clin Psychol 51*, 482-490.

56.   Silbernagel, M. S., Short, S. E., and Ross-Stewart, L. C. (2007) Athletes' use of exercise imagery during weight training., *J Strength Cond Res 21*, 1077-1081.

57.   Jeffery, R. W., Drewnowski, A., Epstein, L. H., Stunkard, A. J., Wilson, G. T., Wing, R. R., and Hill, D. R.

(2000) Long-term maintenance of weight loss: current status., *Health Psychol 19*, 5-16.

58.	Nederkoorn, C., Guerrieri, R., Havermans, R. C., Roefs, A., and Jansen, A. (2009) The interactive effect of hunger and impulsivity on food intake and purchase in a virtual supermarket., *Int J Obes (Lond) 33*, 905-912.

59.	Bacon, L., Stern, J. S., Van Loan, M. D., and Keim, N. L. (2005) Size acceptance and intuitive eating improve health for obese, female chronic dieters., *J Am Diet Assoc 105*, 929-936.

60.	Stice, E., Cameron, R. P., Killen, J. D., Hayward, C., and Taylor, C. B. (1999) Naturalistic weight-reduction efforts prospectively predict growth in relative weight and onset of obesity among female adolescents., *J Consult Clin Psychol 67*, 967-974.

61.	Stice, E., Presnell, K., Shaw, H., and Rohde, P. (2005) Psychological and behavioral risk factors for obesity onset in adolescent girls: a prospective study., *J Consult Clin Psychol 73*, 195-202.

62.	Stote, K. S., Baer, D. J., Spears, K., Paul, D. R., Harris, G. K., Rumpler, W. V., Strycula, P., Najjar, S. S., Ferrucci, L., Ingram, D. K., Longo, D. L., and Mattson, M. P. (2007) A controlled trial of reduced meal frequency without caloric restriction in healthy, normal-weight, middle-aged adults., *Am J Clin Nutr 85*, 981-988.

63.	Kayman, S., Bruvold, W., and Stern, J. S. (1990) Maintenance and relapse after weight loss in women: behavioral aspects., *Am J Clin Nutr 52*, 800-807.

64.	Wyatt, H. R., Grunwald, G. K., Mosca, C. L., Klem, M. L., Wing, R. R., and Hill, J. O. (2002) Long-term weight loss and breakfast in subjects in the National Weight Control Registry., *Obes Res 10*, 78-82.

65.	Geier, A. B., Rozin, P., and Doros, G. (2006) Unit bias. A new heuristic that helps explain the effect of portion size on food intake., *Psychol Sci 17*, 521-525.

66.	McConahy, K. L., Smiciklas-Wright, H., Mitchell, D. C., and Picciano, M. F. (2004) Portion size of common foods predicts energy intake among preschool-aged children., *J Am Diet Assoc 104*, 975-979.

67.   Ledikwe, J. H., Ello-Martin, J. A., and Rolls, B. J. (2005) Portion sizes and the obesity epidemic., *J Nutr 135*, 905-909.

68.   Kant, A. K., and Graubard, B. I. (2004) Eating out in America, 1987-2000: trends and nutritional correlates., *Prev Med 38*, 243-249.

69.   Association, A. D. Tips for eating out. http://www.eatright.org/Public/content.aspx?id=6850. Accessed on 10th November 2011.

70.   Toscos, T., Consolvo, S., and McDonald, D. W. (2011) Barriers to Physical Activity: A Study of Self-Revelation in an Online Community., *J Med Syst*.

71.   Moriarty, D. G., Zack, M. M., and Kobau, R. (2003) The Centers for Disease Control and Prevention's Healthy Days Measures - population tracking of perceived physical and mental health over time., *Health Qual Life Outcomes 1*, 37.

72.   Parschau, L., Richert, J., Koring, M., Ernsting, A., Lippke, S., and Schwarzer, R. (2011) Changes in social-cognitive variables are associated with stage transitions in physical activity., *Health Educ Res*.

73.   Meyer, T., and Broocks, A. (2000) Therapeutic impact of exercise on psychiatric diseases: guidelines for exercise testing and prescription., *Sports Med 30*, 269-279.

74.   van Baak, M. A., van Mil, E., Astrup, A. V., Finer, N., Van Gaal, L. F., Hilsted, J., Kopelman, P. G., Rössner, S., James, W. P., Saris, W. H., and Group, S. S. (2003) Leisure-time activity is an important determinant of long-term weight maintenance after weight loss in the Sibutramine Trial on Obesity Reduction and Maintenance (STORM trial). *Am J Clin Nutr 78*, 209-214.

75.   Caspersen, C. J., Powell, K. E., and Christenson, G. M. (1985) Physical activity, exercise, and physical fitness: definitions and distinctions for health-related research., *Public Health Rep 100*, 126-131.

76.	Jakicic, J. M. (2002) The role of physical activity in prevention and treatment of body weight gain in adults., *J Nutr 132*, 3826S-3829S.
77.	Jakicic, J. M., Wing, R. R., and Winters-Hart, C. (2002) Relationship of physical activity to eating behaviors and weight loss in women., *Med Sci Sports Exerc 34*, 1653-1659.
78.	Hulens, M., Vansant, G., Claessens, A. L., Lysens, R., Muls, E., and Rzewnicki, R. (2002) Health-related quality of life in physically active and sedentary obese women., *Am J Hum Biol 14*, 777-785.
79.	Burke, L. E., Wang, J., and Sevick, M. A. (2011) Self-monitoring in weight loss: a systematic review of the literature., *J Am Diet Assoc 111*, 92-102.
80.	Wing, R. R., and Hill, J. O. (2001) Successful weight loss maintenance., *Annu Rev Nutr 21*, 323-341.
81.	Jeffery, R. W., Bjornson-Benson, W. M., Rosenthal, B. S., Lindquist, R. A., Kurth, C. L., and Johnson, S. L. (1984) Correlates of weight loss and its maintenance over two years of follow-up among middle-aged men., *Prev Med 13*, 155-168.
82.	Bandura, A. (2004) Health promotion by social cognitive means., *Health Educ Behav 31*, 143-164.
83.	Boutelle, K. N., and Kirschenbaum, D. S. (1998) Further support for consistent self-monitoring as a vital component of successful weight control., *Obes Res 6*, 219-224.
84.	Boutelle, K. N., Kirschenbaum, D. S., Baker, R. C., and Mitchell, M. E. (1999) How can obese weight controllers minimize weight gain during the high risk holiday season? By self-monitoring very consistently., *Health Psychol 18*, 364-368.
85.	Baker, R. C., and Kirschenbaum, D. S. (1998) Weight control during the holidays: highly consistent self-monitoring as a potentially useful coping mechanism., *Health Psychol 17*, 367-370.

86.   Helsel, D. L., Jakicic, J. M., and Otto, A. D. (2007) Comparison of techniques for self-monitoring eating and exercise behaviors on weight loss in a correspondence-based intervention., *J Am Diet Assoc 107*, 1807-1810.

87.   Byrne, S., Cooper, Z., and Fairburn, C. (2003) Weight maintenance and relapse in obesity: a qualitative study., *Int J Obes Relat Metab Disord 27*, 955-962.

88.   Carels, R. A., Darby, L. A., Rydin, S., Douglass, O. M., Cacciapaglia, H. M., and O'Brien, W. H. (2005) The relationship between self-monitoring, outcome expectancies, difficulties with eating and exercise, and physical activity and weight loss treatment outcomes., *Ann Behav Med 30*, 182-190.

89.   Bravata, D. M., Smith-Spangler, C., Sundaram, V., Gienger, A. L., Lin, N., Lewis, R., Stave, C. D., Olkin, I., and Sirard, J. R. (2007) Using pedometers to increase physical activity and improve health: a systematic review., *JAMA 298*, 2296-2304.

90.   Araiza, P., Hewes, H., Gashetewa, C., Vella, C. A., and Burge, M. R. (2006) Efficacy of a pedometer-based physical activity program on parameters of diabetes control in type 2 diabetes mellitus., *Metabolism 55*, 1382-1387.

91.   Schneider, P. L., Bassett, D. R., Thompson, D. L., Pronk, N. P., and Bielak, K. M. (2006) Effects of a 10,000 steps per day goal in overweight adults., *Am J Health Promot 21*, 85-89.

92.   Eastep, E., Beveridge, S., Eisenman, P., Ransdell, L., and Shultz, B. (2004) Does augmented feedback from pedometers increase adults' walking behavior?, *Percept Mot Skills 99*, 392-402.

93.   VanWormer, J. J., Martinez, A. M., Martinson, B. C., Crain, A. L., Benson, G. A., Cosentino, D. L., and Pronk, N. P. (2009) Self-weighing promotes weight loss for obese adults., *Am J Prev Med 36*, 70-73.

94.   Linde, J. A., Jeffery, R. W., French, S. A., Pronk, N. P., and Boyle, R. G. (2005) Self-weighing in weight gain

prevention and weight loss trials., *Ann Behav Med 30*, 210-216.

95.	Yon, B. A., Johnson, R. K., Harvey-Berino, J., Gold, B. C., and Howard, A. B. (2007) Personal digital assistants are comparable to traditional diaries for dietary self-monitoring during a weight loss program., *J Behav Med 30*, 165-175.

96.	Kuijer, R., de Ridder, D., Ouwehand, C., Houx, B., and van den Bos, R. (2008) Dieting as a case of behavioural decision making. Does self-control matter?, *Appetite 51*, 506-511.

97.	Just, D. R., and Payne, C. R. (2009) Obesity: can behavioral economics help?, *Ann Behav Med 38 Suppl 1*, S47-55.

98.	Ferguson, K. J., Brink, P. J., Wood, M., and Koop, P. M. (1992) Characteristics of successful dieters as measured by guided interview responses and Restraint Scale scores., *J Am Diet Assoc 92*, 1119-1121.

99.	Rotter, J. B. (1966) Generalized expectancies for internal versus external control of reinforcement., *Psychol Monogr 80*, 1-28.

100.	Holt, C. L., Clark, E. M., and Kreuter, M. W. (2001) Weight locus of control and weight-related attitudes and behaviors in an overweight population., *Addict Behav 26*, 329-340.

101.	Ogden, J. (2000) The correlates of long-term weight loss: a group comparison study of obesity., *Int J Obes Relat Metab Disord 24*, 1018-1025.

102.	Zijlstra, H., Boeije, H. R., Larsen, J. K., van Ramshorst, B., and Geenen, R. (2009) Patients' explanations for unsuccessful weight loss after laparoscopic adjustable gastric banding (LAGB). *Patient Educ Couns 75*, 108-113.

103.	Carels, R. A., Konrad, K., Young, K. M., Darby, L. A., Coit, C., Clayton, A. M., and Oemig, C. K. (2008) Taking control of your personal eating and exercise environment: a weight maintenance program., *Eat Behav 9*, 228-237.

104.   Administration, T. U. S. F. a. D. (Accessed: 10/03/2011) http://www.fda.gov/Food/LabelingNutrition/ConsumerInformation/ucm078889.htm.

105.   Kruger, J., Blanck, H. M., and Gillespie, C. (2008) Dietary practices, dining out behavior, and physical activity correlates of weight loss maintenance., *Prev Chronic Dis 5*, A11.

106.   Kruger, J., Blanck, H. M., and Gillespie, C. (2006) Dietary and physical activity behaviors among adults successful at weight loss maintenance., *Int J Behav Nutr Phys Act 3*, 17.

107.   Gallagher, K. I., Jakicic, J. M., Napolitano, M. A., and Marcus, B. H. (2006) Psychosocial factors related to physical activity and weight loss in overweight women., *Med Sci Sports Exerc 38*, 971-980.

108.   Verheijden, M. W., Bakx, J. C., van Weel, C., Koelen, M. A., and van Staveren, W. A. (2005) Role of social support in lifestyle-focused weight management interventions., *Eur J Clin Nutr 59 Suppl 1*, S179-186.

109.   Perri, M. G., Sears, S. F., and Clark, J. E. (1993) Strategies for improving maintenance of weight loss. Toward a continuous care model of obesity management., *Diabetes Care 16*, 200-209.

110.   DePue, J. D., Clark, M. M., Ruggiero, L., Medeiros, M. L., and Pera, V. (1995) Maintenance of weight loss: a needs assessment., *Obes Res 3*, 241-248.

111.   Hindle, L., and Carpenter, C. (2011) An exploration of the experiences and perceptions of people who have maintained weight loss., *J Hum Nutr Diet 24*, 342-350.

112.   Andrews, G. (1997) Intimate saboteurs., *Obes Surg 7*, 445-448.

113.   Wing, R. R., and Jeffery, R. W. (1999) Benefits of recruiting participants with friends and increasing social support for weight loss and maintenance., *J Consult Clin Psychol 67*, 132-138.

114.   Wagner, J., Burg, M., and Sirois, B. (2004) Social support and the transtheoretical model: Relationship of social support to smoking cessation stage, decisional balance, process use, and temptation., *Addict Behav 29*, 1039-1043.
115.   Hwang, K. O., Farheen, K., Johnson, C. W., Thomas, E. J., Barnes, A. S., and Bernstam, E. V. (2007) Quality of weight loss advice on internet forums., *Am J Med 120*, 604-609.
116.   White, M., and Dorman, S. M. (2001) Receiving social support online: implications for health education., *Health Educ Res 16*, 693-707.
117.   Tanis, M. (2008) Health-related on-line forums: what's the big attraction?, *J Health Commun 13*, 698-714.
118.   Johnson, F., and Wardle, J. (2011) The association between weight loss and engagement with a web-based food and exercise diary in a commercial weight loss programme: a retrospective analysis., *Int J Behav Nutr Phys Act 8*, 83.
119.   Spalding, K. L., Arner, E., Westermark, P. O., Bernard, S., Buchholz, B. A., Bergmann, O., Blomqvist, L., Hoffstedt, J., Näslund, E., Britton, T., Concha, H., Hassan, M., Rydén, M., Frisén, J., and Arner, P. (2008) Dynamics of fat cell turnover in humans., *Nature 453*, 783-787.
120.   Agriculture, U. S. D. o. Dietary Guidelines for Americans   2010. http://www.health.gov/dietaryguidelines/dga2010/DietaryGuidelines2010.pdf. Accessed on 21st November 2011.
121.   Agriculture, U. S. D. o. Dietary Guidelines for Americans 2010. www.dietaryguidelines.gov. Accessed on 21st November 2011.
122.   "food." *Encyclopædia Britannica. Encyclopædia Britannica Online.* Encyclopædia Britannica Inc., W. N. **h. w. b. c. E. t. f.**
123.   Rolls, B. J. (1995) Carbohydrates, fats, and satiety., *Am J Clin Nutr 61*, 960S-967S.

124.   Control., C. f. D. Carbohydrates.http://www.cdc.gov/nutrition/everyone/basics/carbs.html Accessed on 8Th of November 2011.

125.   Control., C. f. D. Proteins. http://www.cdc.gov/nutrition/everyone/basics/protein.html. Accessed on 20th of November 2011.

126.   Josse, A. R., Atkinson, S. A., Tarnopolsky, M. A., and Phillips, S. M. (2011) Increased consumption of dairy foods and protein during diet- and exercise-induced weight loss promotes fat mass loss and lean mass gain in overweight and obese premenopausal women., *J Nutr 141*, 1626-1634.

127.   Micha, R., and Mozaffarian, D. (2009) Trans fatty acids: effects on metabolic syndrome, heart disease and diabetes., *Nat Rev Endocrinol 5*, 335-344.

128.   Control., C. f. D. Vitamins and Minerals. http://www.cdc.gov/nutrition/everyone/basics/vitamins/. Accessed on 8Th of November 2011.

129.   encyclopedia, W.-t. f. Addiction, http://en.wikipedia.org/wiki/Addiction.

130.   Del Parigi, A., Chen, K., Salbe, A. D., Reiman, E. M., and Tataranni, P. A. (2003) Are we addicted to food?, *Obes Res 11*, 493-495.

131.   Kalivas, P. W., and Volkow, N. D. (2005) The neural basis of addiction: a pathology of motivation and choice., *Am J Psychiatry 162*, 1403-1413.

132.   Kelley, A. E., Baldo, B. A., and Pratt, W. E. (2005) A proposed hypothalamic-thalamic-striatal axis for the integration of energy balance, arousal, and food reward., *J Comp Neurol 493*, 72-85.

133.   Saelens, B. E., and Epstein, L. H. (1996) Reinforcing value of food in obese and non-obese women., *Appetite 27*, 41-50.

134.   Johnson, W. G. (1974) Effect of cue prominence and subject weight on human food-directed performance., *J Pers Soc Psychol 29*, 843-848.

135.   Wang, G. J., Volkow, N. D., Logan, J., Pappas, N. R., Wong, C. T., Zhu, W., Netusil, N., and Fowler, J. S. (2001) Brain dopamine and obesity., *Lancet 357*, 354-357.
136.   Mokdad, A. H., Marks, J. S., Stroup, D. F., and Gerberding, J. L. (2004) Actual causes of death in the United States, 2000., *JAMA 291*, 1238-1245.
137.   Elliott, S. S., Keim, N. L., Stern, J. S., Teff, K., and Havel, P. J. (2002) Fructose, weight gain, and the insulin resistance syndrome., *Am J Clin Nutr 76*, 911-922.
138.   Howard, B. V., and Wylie-Rosett, J. (2002) Sugar and cardiovascular disease: A statement for healthcare professionals from the Committee on Nutrition of the Council on Nutrition, Physical Activity, and Metabolism of the American Heart Association., *Circulation 106*, 523-527.
139.   Ludwig, D. S., Peterson, K. E., and Gortmaker, S. L. (2001) Relation between consumption of sugar-sweetened drinks and childhood obesity: a prospective, observational analysis., *Lancet 357*, 505-508.
140.   Johnson, R. J., and Murray, R. (2010) Fructose, exercise, and health., *Curr Sports Med Rep 9*, 253-258.
141.   Lê, K. A., and Tappy, L. (2006) Metabolic effects of fructose., *Curr Opin Clin Nutr Metab Care 9*, 469-475.
142.   Sato, Y., Ito, T., Udaka, N., Kanisawa, M., Noguchi, Y., Cushman, S. W., and Satoh, S. (1996) Immunohistochemical localization of facilitated-diffusion glucose transporters in rat pancreatic islets., *Tissue Cell 28*, 637-643.
143.   Vilsbøll, T., Krarup, T., Madsbad, S., and Holst, J. J. (2003) Both GLP-1 and GIP are insulinotropic at basal and postprandial glucose levels and contribute nearly equally to the incretin effect of a meal in healthy subjects., *Regul Pept 114*, 115-121.
144.   Schwartz, M. W., Woods, S. C., Porte, D., Seeley, R. J., and Baskin, D. G. (2000) Central nervous system control of food intake., *Nature 404*, 661-671.
145.   Saad, M. F., Khan, A., Sharma, A., Michael, R., Riad-Gabriel, M. G., Boyadjian, R., Jinagouda, S. D., Steil, G. M.,

and Kamdar, V. (1998) Physiological insulinemia acutely modulates plasma leptin., *Diabetes 47*, 544-549.

146.   Teff, K. L., Elliott, S. S., Tschöp, M., Kieffer, T. J., Rader, D., Heiman, M., Townsend, R. R., Keim, N. L., D'Alessio, D., and Havel, P. J. (2004) Dietary fructose reduces circulating insulin and leptin, attenuates postprandial suppression of ghrelin, and increases triglycerides in women., *J Clin Endocrinol Metab 89*, 2963-2972.

147.   Bray, G. A., Nielsen, S. J., and Popkin, B. M. (2004) Consumption of high-fructose corn syrup in beverages may play a role in the epidemic of obesity., *Am J Clin Nutr 79*, 537-543.

148.   JONHNSON, R., and GOWER, T. The Sugar Fix:The High-Fructose Fallout That Is Making You Fat and Sick (2008).

149.   Marriott, B. P., Cole, N., and Lee, E. (2009) National estimates of dietary fructose intake increased from 1977 to 2004 in the United States., *J Nutr 139*, 1228S-1235S.

150.   Phelan, S., Wyatt, H. R., Hill, J. O., and Wing, R. R. (2006) Are the eating and exercise habits of successful weight losers changing?, *Obesity (Silver Spring) 14*, 710-716.

151.   Jonnalagadda, S. S., Harnack, L., Liu, R. H., McKeown, N., Seal, C., Liu, S., and Fahey, G. C. (2011) Putting the whole grain puzzle together: health benefits associated with whole grains--summary of American Society for Nutrition 2010 Satellite Symposium, *J Nutr 141*, 1011S-1022S.

152.   Liu, S., Willett, W. C., Manson, J. E., Hu, F. B., Rosner, B., and Colditz, G. (2003) Relation between changes in intakes of dietary fiber and grain products and changes in weight and development of obesity among middle-aged women, *Am J Clin Nutr 78*, 920-927.

153.   Koh-Banerjee, P., Franz, M., Sampson, L., Liu, S., Jacobs, D. R., Spiegelman, D., Willett, W., and Rimm, E. (2004) Changes in whole-grain, bran, and cereal fiber

consumption in relation to 8-y weight gain among men, *Am J Clin Nutr 80*, 1237-1245.

154.   Fulgoni, V. L., Dreher, M., and Davenport, A. J. (2013) Avocado consumption is associated with better diet quality and nutrient intake, and lower metabolic syndrome risk in US adults: results from the National Health and Nutrition Examination Survey (NHANES) 2001-2008, *Nutr J 12*, 1.

155.   Basu, A., Rhone, M., and Lyons, T. J. (2010) Berries: emerging impact on cardiovascular health, *Nutr Rev 68*, 168-177.

156.   Wu, F., Yang, N., Touré, A., Jin, Z., and Xu, X. (2013) Germinated brown rice and its role in human health, *Crit Rev Food Sci Nutr 53*, 451-463.

157.   Imam, M. U., Azmi, N. H., Bhanger, M. I., Ismail, N., and Ismail, M. (2012) Antidiabetic properties of germinated brown rice: a systematic review, *Evid Based Complement Alternat Med 2012*, 816501.

158.   Vander Wal, J. S., Gupta, A., Khosla, P., and Dhurandhar, N. V. (2008) Egg breakfast enhances weight loss, *Int J Obes (Lond) 32*, 1545-1551.

159.   Pearce, K. L., Clifton, P. M., and Noakes, M. (2011) Egg consumption as part of an energy-restricted high-protein diet improves blood lipid and blood glucose profiles in individuals with type 2 diabetes, *Br J Nutr 105*, 584-592.

160.   Sabaté, J., Oda, K., and Ros, E. (2010) Nut consumption and blood lipid levels: a pooled analysis of 25 intervention trials, *Arch Intern Med 170*, 821-827.

161.   Sabaté, J., and Ang, Y. (2009) Nuts and health outcomes: new epidemiologic evidence, *Am J Clin Nutr 89*, 1643S-1648S.

162.   Wang, S. Y., Huang, W. C., Liu, C. C., Wang, M. F., Ho, C. S., Huang, W. P., Hou, C. C., Chuang, H. L., and Huang, C. C. (2012) Pumpkin (Cucurbita moschata) fruit extract improves physical fatigue and exercise performance in mice, *Molecules 17*, 11864-11876.

163.   Yoshinari, O., Sato, H., and Igarashi, K. (2009) Anti-diabetic effects of pumpkin and its components, trigonelline and nicotinic acid, on Goto-Kakizaki rats, *Biosci Biotechnol Biochem 73*, 1033-1041.

164.   Chan, J. Y., Yuen, A. C., Chan, R. Y., and Chan, S. W. (2012) A Review of the Cardiovascular Benefits and Antioxidant Properties of Allicin, *Phytother Res.*

165.   Whiting, S., Derbyshire, E., and Tiwari, B. K. (2012) Capsaicinoids and capsinoids. A potential role for weight management? A systematic review of the evidence, *Appetite 59*, 341-348.

166.   Mahmoud, R. H., and Elnour, W. A. (2013) Comparative evaluation of the efficacy of ginger and orlistat on obesity management, pancreatic lipase and liver peroxisomal catalase enzyme in male albino rats, *Eur Rev Med Pharmacol Sci 17*, 75-83.

167.   Khan, A., Safdar, M., Ali Khan, M. M., Khattak, K. N., and Anderson, R. A. (2003) Cinnamon improves glucose and lipids of people with type 2 diabetes, *Diabetes Care 26*, 3215-3218.

168.   Hlebowicz, J., Darwiche, G., Björgell, O., and Almér, L. O. (2007) Effect of cinnamon on postprandial blood glucose, gastric emptying, and satiety in healthy subjects, *Am J Clin Nutr 85*, 1552-1556.

169.   Svalina, S. S., and Webb, J. R. (2011) Forgiveness and health among people in outpatient physical therapy., *Disabil Rehabil.*

170.   Worthington, E. L., van Oyen Witvliet, C., Lerner, A. J., and Scherer, M. (2005) Forgiveness in health research and medical practice., *Explore (NY) 1*, 169-176.

171.   Roberts, C., Troop, N., Connan, F., Treasure, J., and Campbell, I. C. (2007) The effects of stress on body weight: biological and psychological predictors of change in BMI., *Obesity (Silver Spring) 15*, 3045-3055.

172.   Clinic., M. Overcoming weight loss setbacks. http://www.mayoclinic.com/health/weight-loss/WT00021. Accessed on 1st December 2011.